全国中医药行业高等教育"十四五"创新教材

中医英语口语教程

（供中医学等专业用）

主 编 胡双全 罗 茜

全国百佳图书出版单位
中国中医药出版社
·北 京·

图书在版编目（CIP）数据

中医英语口语教程 / 胡双全，罗茜主编 . —北京：
中国中医药出版社，2023.12
全国中医药行业高等教育"十四五"创新教材
ISBN 978-7-5132-8592-6

Ⅰ . ①中… Ⅱ . ①胡… ②罗… Ⅲ . 中国医药学—
英语—中医学院—教材 Ⅳ . ① R2

中国国家版本馆 CIP 数据核字（2023）第 228772 号

中国中医药出版社出版
北京经济技术开发区科创十三街 31 号院二区 8 号楼
邮政编码 100176
传真 010－64405721
廊坊市佳艺印务有限公司印刷
各地新华书店经销

开本 787×1092 1/16 印张 8.25 字数 270 千字
2023 年 12 月第 1 版 2023 年 12 月第 1 次印刷
书号 ISBN 978－7－5132－8592－6

定价 39.00 元
网址 www.cptcm.com

服 务 热 线 010-64405510
购 书 热 线 010-89535836
维 权 打 假 010-64405753

微信服务号 zgzyycbs
微商城网址 https://kdt.im/LIdUGr
官 方 微 博 http://e.weibo.com/cptcm
天猫旗舰店网址 https://zgzyycbs.tmall.com

如有印装质量问题请与本社出版部联系（010－64405510）

全国中医药行业高等教育"十四五"创新教材

《中医英语口语教程》编委会

主　　审　单宝枝（中国中医药出版社有限公司）

　　　　　王银泉（南京农业大学）

主　　编　胡双全（江西中医药大学）

　　　　　罗　茜（江西中医药大学）

副 主 编　余　静（江西中医药大学）

　　　　　艾卫平（江西中医药大学）

　　　　　刘　成（江西中医药大学）

　　　　　杨具荣（江西中医药大学）

　　　　　肖笑飞（江西中医药大学）

编　　委　（按姓氏笔画排序）

　　　　　万莉莉（江西中医药大学）

　　　　　王小芳（江西中医药大学）

　　　　　任俊伟（江西中医药大学）

　　　　　周　媛（江西中医药大学）

　　　　　赵永红（江西中医药大学）

　　　　　胡奇军（江西中医药大学）

　　　　　涂宇明（江西中医药大学）

　　　　　谌志远（江西中医药大学）

　　　　　韩　露（江西中医药大学）

　　　　　熊　展（江西中医药大学）

编写说明

　　随着国际医学技术交流的日益频繁，医学英语已成为我国医务工作者了解与学习国外医学前沿知识、弘扬中医学所必须掌握的一门语言交流工具。21 世纪以来，我国各中医药院十分重视中医英语的教学，相继开设了中医类专门用途的英语课程。

　　为了提高中医药院校毕业生在工作场合、学术场合运用英语开展交流沟通的能力，我们结合江西地区中医药事业发展现状，特此编写了《中医英语口语教程》，以满足相关读者市场需求。本教材可以帮助学习者掌握用英语交流中医知识、理论和中医疗法，传播中医文化的能力，同时本教材也重视立德树人，坚持育人与育德的有机统一，融入了中医核心价值观，以培养学生对中医药文化的自信。

　　本教材的内容集中于中医医学生必须掌握的中医医学英语知识，以及这些知识点在日常就医、学术交流、国际交流等场合中的应用。本教材在内容设计上涵盖了医学院校学生英语学习的基本需求，既包括了中医基础医学方面的英语，也包括了临床医学方面的英语；既有医学专业英语，又有药学专业英语；还包括医学生和医务工作者所需的科研英语。因此，本教材可供中医院校按需使用。

　　为使学生学习医学英语时有整体观念，本教材以中医基础理论为编写大纲，内容涵盖阴阳、五行、藏象、四诊、八纲辨证等。

　　本教材根据中医话题分为 12 章，每章基本由五部分组成：① Lead-in Questions。此部分设置了一些导入性的问题，目的是启发学生思维，导入课程内容。② Useful Expressions。此部分介绍了和话题相关的单词、短语、句子表达等语料素材，帮助学生积累话题表达所需的语言元素。③ Model Dialogues。此部分提供的是虚拟场景的对话，目的是帮助学生了解中医在日常生活中的运用，学生应熟读对话。④ Oral Practice。此部分为口语训练，设置了场景对话、中医故事讲述、团队项目、深入阅读及回答问题等环节，这些口语练习可以帮助学习者学以致用，巩固所学知识理论。⑤ Creative Oral Activity。这一部分具有地方特色，设计了一些与江西本地医药和创新创业相关的话题，目的是激发学生讨论的兴趣，培养其创造性思维，同时训练其口语表达能力。

本教材的编写分工如下。胡双全负责编写第一章～第三章，罗茜负责编写第四章、第五章，杨具荣负责编写第六章，周媛负责编写第七章，任俊伟负责编写第八章，余静负责编写第九章、第十章，刘成负责编写第十一章、第十二章。本教材的文字编辑和审核工作分工如下：赵永红负责第一章、第二章，涂宇明负责第三章、第四章，万莉莉负责第五章、第六章，熊展负责第七章、第八章，韩露负责第九章、第十章，胡奇军负责第七章，王小芳、谌志远负责第十二章。艾卫平负责第一章～第六章的校对工作，肖笑飞负责第七章～第十二章的校对工作。本教材第一章～第六章的主审工作由中国中医药出版社有限公司的单宝枝教授负责，第七章～第十二章的主审工作由南京农业大学的王银泉教授负责，在此对两位主审表示衷心的感谢！

《中医英语口语教程》编委会

2023 年 12 月

Catalog

Chapter One

The History of Traditional Chinese Medicine (TCM)

Learning Objectives

In this chapter you will learn:
● How to introduce stories related with TCM;
● How to introduce famous doctors of Chinese medicine and their works;
● Conduct a series of speaking activities;
● Complete a creative oral task.

I Lead-in Questions

1. Can you tell any tales about TCM?

2. What is the importance of TCM to Chinese people?

3. Can you name some famous TCM doctors in Chinese history and their literature works?

II Useful Expressions

New Words and Phrases

1. antiquity /ænˈtɪkwəti/ *n.* (pl. -ies) the ancient past, especially the times of the Greeks and Romans 古代

2. acupuncture /ˈækjupʌŋktʃə (r)/ *n.* a Chinese method of treating pain and illness using special thin needles which are pushed into the skin in particular parts of the body 针刺疗法

3. moxibustion /ˌmɒksɪˈbʌstʃən/ *n.* a method of treatment, originally in Chinese medicine, in which a moxa is burned on the skin 灸法

4. cupping therapy 拔罐

5. skin scraping /ˈskreɪpɪŋ/ 刮痧

6. herb /hɜːb/ *n.* a plant whose leaves, flowers or seeds are used to flavour food, in medicines or for their pleasant smell 药草

7. physician /fɪˈzɪʃn/ *n.* a doctor, especially one who is a specialist in general medicine and not surgery（尤指）内科医生

8. monograph /ˈmɒnəɡrɑːf/ *n.* a detailed written study of a single subject, usually in the form of a short book 专论；专著

9. extant /ekˈstænt/ *adj.* (of sth very old) still in existence 尚存的；现存的

10. materia medica /məˈtɪərɪə ˈmɛdɪkə/ *n.* the body of remedial substances used in the practice of medicine 本草

11. anesthesia /ˌænɪsˈθiːzɪə/ *n.* 麻醉

12. pathology /pəˈθɒlədʒi/ *n.* the scientific study of diseases 病理学

13. exogenous /ekˈsɒdʒənəs/ *adj.* having a cause that is outside the body 外源性的

14. purgation /pɜːˈɡeɪʃən/ *n.* the act of purging or state of being purged; purification 通便，催泻

15. pestilence /ˈpɛstɪləns/ *n.* any disease that spreads quickly and kills a lot of people 瘟疫

16. infectious /ɪnˈfekʃəs/ *adj.* an infectious disease can be passed easily from one person to another, especially through the air they breathe 传染性的

17. epidemic /epɪˈdemɪk/ *n.* a large number of cases of a particular disease happening at the same time in a particular community 流行病

18. etiology /iːtɪˈɒlədʒɪ/ *n.* the etiology of a disease or a problem is the study of its causes 病原学

19. meditation /ˌmedɪˈteɪʃn/ *n.* the practice of thinking deeply in silence, especially for religious reasons or in order to make your mind calm 冥想；沉思

20. massage /ˈmæsɑːʒ/ *n.* the action of rubbing and pressing a person's body with the hands to reduce pain in the muscles and joints 按摩

21. healthy *qi* 正气

22. dietetic /ˌdaɪəˈtetɪk/ therapy 食疗

23. physiotherapy /ˌfɪziəʊˈθerəpi/ *n.* the treatment of disease, injury or weakness in the joints or muscles by exercises, massage and the use of light and heat 理疗

24. radiotherapy /ˌreɪdiəʊˈθerəpi/ *n.* the treatment of disease by radiation 放射疗法

25. chemotherapy /ˌkiːməʊˈθerəpi/ *n.* the treatment of disease, especially cancer, with the use of chemical substances 化疗

26. health-care /ˈhelθ ker/ 保健

27. incise /ɪnˈsaɪz/ *vt.* to cut words, designs, etc. into a surface 切入

28. porcelain /ˈpɔːsəlɪn/ *n.* a hard white shiny substance made by baking clay and

used for making delicate cups, plates and decorative objects 瓷；瓷器

29. calabash /ˈkæləbæʃ/ *n.* 葫芦果

Sentence Patterns

● How to introduce the development of Chinese medicine and their works

1. The origin of TCM (traditional Chinese medicine) can be traced back to remote antiquity in China.

2. Traditional Chinese medicine is created by Chinese people. It is a subject that studies human physiology, pathology, treatment and prevention of diseases.

3. Traditional Chinese medicine is the summary of the experience and knowledge from ancient Chinese people fighting against diseases.

4. The acupuncture of TCM has good reputation in the global world.

5. Based on the theory of yin and yang and five elements, traditional Chinese medicine regards human body as the unity of *qi*, physical body and spirit.

6. TCM applies the four diagnostic methods to inspect patients.

7. Due to the "Belt and Road Initiative", Chinese authorities are paying more attention to the development of TCM.

8. During the period of fighting against COVID-19 in 2020, Chinese medicine has played an important role in the treatment.

9. TCM has now been widely recognized and applied in different countries.

● How to introduce famous doctors of Chinese medicine and their works

1. The legend of Shennong tasted a hundred kinds of herbs in a day, and he experienced seventy kinds of poisons shows the devotion of Shennong to the development of TCM.

2. In the late Eastern Han Dynasty (25-220 AD), the eminent physician Zhang Zhongjing wrote a book called *Classic on Medical Problems* based upon the *Huangdi's Internal Classic.*

3. The *Huangdi's Internal Classic* explained the laws of life and the unity of the body with the natural world.

4. The *Essentials from the Golden Cabinet* used the theory of disease processes in the *zang* and *fu* to formulate the classification and diagnosis of diseases.

5. *Shennong's Classic of Materia Medica* is the oldest monograph extant in China. This work summarized descriptions of 365 distinct Chinese herbs, and classified them into three grades: superior, medium and inferior. It systematically summed up the knowledge and experiences of people in the Qin and Han dynasties, and also exerted important influence on the subsequent development in the field of Chinese materia medica.

6. Zhang Zhongjing, a famous physician in the Eastern Han Dynasty proposed eight

kinds of treatment methods based on "Eight Principles" (yin and yang, exterior and interior, deficiency and excess, cold and heat) .

7. Hua Tuo was a famous doctor in surgery and anesthesia. He invented the "Five-animal Exercise" , a kind of body-building exercise from imitating the movements of five kinds animals such as tiger, deer, bear, ape and bird.

8. Huangfu Mi compiled his *A-B Classic of Acupuncture and Moxibustion*, the oldest extant monograph in China on acupuncture and moxibustion.

9. Wang Shuhe compiled the book *Pulse Classic* which summarized the 24 kinds of pulse manifestations relating to the principal diseases and systematized the theory of the pulse.

10. During the Sui Dynasty (581-618 AD), Chao Yuanfang and his colleagues compiled their *Treatise on the Causes and Manifestations of Various Diseases*. This was TCM's first monograph of pathology.

● TCM Literature Works

English Titles	Chinese Titles	Authors
Huangdi's Internal Classic	《黄帝内经》	Unknown
Classic on Difficult Medical Problems	《难经》	qin Yueren
Treatise on Cold-Attack and Miscellaneous Diseases	《伤寒杂病论》	Zhang Zhongjing
Essentials from the Golden Cabinet	《金匮要略》	Zhang Zhongjing
Shennong's Classic of Materia Medica	《神农本草经》	Unknown
Pulse Classic	《脉经》	Wang Shuhe
A-B Classic of Acupuncture and Moxibustion	《针灸甲乙经》	Huangfu Mi
Treatise on the Causes and Manifestations of Various Diseases	《诸病源候论》	Chao Yuanfang
Newly Revised Materia Medica	《新修本草》	Su Jing etc.
Prescriptions Worth a Thousand Gold Pieces for Emergency	《备急千金药方》	Sun Simiao
Complete Effective Prescriptions for Women	《妇人良方》	Chen Ziming
Key to Medicines and Patterns of Children's Diseases	《小儿药证直诀》	Qian Yi
Compendium of Materia Medica	《本草纲目》	Li Shizhen

● How to introduce different medical schools and their propositions:

(1) Liu Wansu— the school of cooling. He emphasized the usage of herbal drugs cold and cool in nature because the "six exogenous" factors all arise from fire and "five emotions in excess would turn into fire".

(2) Zhang Congzheng— the school of purgation. He believed that all diseases were caused by "evil factors" . Once the pathogenic factors were expelled, the normal conditions of the body would naturally be restored.

(3) Li Gao— the school of strengthening the spleen and stomach. He thought that

diseases, apart from external causes, were mainly brought about by internal injury of the spleen and stomach, and advocating cure by building up and regulating the spleen and stomach.

(4) Zhu Danxi— the school of nourishing yin. He said "the body often has more than enough yang but not enough yin". So, he emphasized the principle of nourishing yin and reducing fire for treatment of diseases.

(5) Traditional Chinese medicine is the treasure of Chinese civilization. We should promote the integration of production, teaching and research, the industrialization and modernization of Chinese medicine, and bring the Chinese medicine into the world.

(6) *Treatise on Pestilence* was written by Wu Youke in the Ming Dynasty. He was the first person who put forward "pestilential *qi*" and believed that the infectious epidemic diseases were caused neither by wind, cold, summer heat nor damp, but a kind of evil *qi* in the nature which invaded the body through the mouth and nose rather than from the body surface. His idea made a breakthrough in the development of etiology for infectious febrile diseases.

III Model Dialogues

Conversation 1

Lucy: Hi, Li Ming. What is the thick book you are reading?

Li Ming: I am reading *Huangdi's Internal Classic,* one of the four greatest TCM classic literature works.

Lucy: Amazing. I am very interested in Chinese medicine, and I've heard of the book before, but honestly I know nothing about it. Could you tell me something about it?

Li Ming: Well, the book can be divided into two volumes— *Su Wen* (Plain Conversation) and *Ling Shu* (Spiritual Pivot), each containing 81 chapters, so that's 162 chapters in total.

Lucy: Wow, that is truly a big book to read.

Li Ming: Yes, it's a comprehensive book which contains theories on yin and yang, pulse manifestation, visceral manifestation, channels and collaterals, syndrome differentiation, health preservation, etiology, etc.

Lucy: So, the book is just like an encyclopedia on Chinese medicine.

Li Ming: Yes, you can say that again. The book puts forward a complete medical system for TCM and has laid the foundation for human physiology, pathology, diagnosis and treatment in traditional Chinese medicine.

Lucy: Can I borrow your book? I can't wait to read it.

Li Ming: Of course, you can. I mean you can have my book, but it might be difficult for you to understand. The book is written in ancient Chinese style, and it is even difficult for me, let alone a foreigner like you. But don't worry , you can read the express edition.

Lucy: Good idea. Where can I have the express edition?

Li Ming: You can borrow it from the school library.

Conversation 2

Jason: I was told that there are many famous TCM doctors in ancient times in China, especially during the Jin and Yuan Dynasties.

Li Ming: Yes, there were four representative TCM doctors during that time, and they are called The Great Doctors in Jin and Yuan Dynasties.

Jason: I know, one of the doctors is called Liu Wansu, and he propounded the theory of fire-heat, right?

Li Ming: Yes, he believed that six kinds of climatic factors could become internal fire and most diseases were caused by fire and heat, so he preferred using medicines which are cold and cool by nature when treating diseases, and for this reason he was labeled as the school of cold-cool.

Jason: Wow, unbelievable! You are almost like an expert on TCM.

Li Ming: You flattered me. I am a layman of TCM. I read a book about Liu Wansu last week. It said that Liu was smart when he was a child. When he was 25 years old, his mother was badly sick, and he tried to send for a doctor for 3 times, but in vain and his mother passed away shortly after that. Due to this incident, Liu made up his mind to study on Chinese medicine.

Jason: I feel sorry for his loss. So what about other three doctors?

Li Ming: They are Zhang Congzheng, Li Gao and Zhu Zhenheng.

Jason: Can you tell me more about them?

Li Ming: Come on, Jason. I know you are interested in them, but it's a long story to go. Maybe we can sit down in a cafe and talk about them over a coffee.

Jason: Yeah, that is a good idea. My treat.

IV Oral Practice

Situational Dialogues

Work in teams and make up dialogues based on the following situations.

Situation 1

Lucy heard that TCM has a history of over 5000 years, and she has always been interested in TCM. One day, when she was visiting the museum, she was attracted by *Bianshi*— the stone for treatment in TCM. It made her surprised that ancient Chinese people could use stone to dispel disease. You play the role of a guide working in the museum and tell her more about *Bianshi* in TCM.

Situation 2

You are a guide and you are now showing a group of American tourists around in a TCM museum. On the walls, there are many pictures of famous TCM doctors in ancient China, as well as some doctors who made great contributions in the fight against COVID-19, such as Zhong Nanshan, Zhang Boli and Chen Wei. You are introducing those doctors to the tourists.

Situation 3

During the fight against the pandemic (coronavirus), TCM proved to have effective curing function, thus attracting the attention from all over the world. You are invited to make a speech on the future of TCM in a foreign university.

Story-retelling

Cue Words

(1) 杏树   apricot trees
(2) 重病   serious disease
(3) 小病   minor illness
(4) 粮仓   barn
(5) 谷物   grain
(6) 取之于民，用之于民   take from people and use it for people
(7) 盘缠   travelling expense
(8) 神仙   immortal
(9) 救死扶伤   heal the wounded and rescue the dying

杏 林

三国时期，吴国有个很有名气的民间医师叫董奉。此人具有高明的医术、高尚的医德，乐做善事，施恩从不图回报。他在庐山南麓定居后，守着大片山地不种田，而是给人治病，且不收分文。病人及亲属想表达感激之情，董奉就提出，如果病治好了，患者就在山地栽杏树：病重治愈者，种五棵；病轻治愈者，种一棵。如此多年，共栽下杏树十万多株，成了一片郁郁葱葱的大杏林。每年杏子成熟季节，硕果累累。为处理这些杏子，董奉就在杏林中建了一个粮仓。他告诉人们，如果有想买杏子的，不必告诉他，可以谷物换杏，只要把带来的谷子倒入粮仓，自己取回相当数量杏子即可。董医师每年用杏子换来许多谷子，他坚持取之于民，用之于民，把谷子用来救济周围的贫苦百姓，接济来庐山旅行而断了盘缠的人。据说，每年经他救济的人在两万以上。知道这些神奇事情的人认定董奉是上天派下凡的神仙，是专门来救死扶伤、解危济困的。从此，"杏林"一词也就流传衍变为中医药的代名词了。

Group Task

Task 1

Talk about the phenomenon of "Bare-foot Doctors" existed in 1960s and 1970s in China. Please search for information about this special phenomenon in China and hold a discussion with your teammates. Write a report to summarize your team discussion.

Task 2

Work with your teammates, searching for information about famous doctors of Chinese medicine in the local area. Each group will assign a representative to report what will be found.

Reading and Question Answering

TCM: Chinese Medicine with a Long History

Traditional Chinese Medicine (TCM) has a history of over 5000 years, it can be traced back to remote antiquity. In a long course of struggling against diseases, TCM evolved into a unique and integrated theoretical system of TCM. Besides, it is regarded as a unique traditional Chinese culture.

More than 2,000 years ago, The *Huangdi's Internal Classic* (*Huang Di Nei Jing*) came into being. The medical classic is made up of two parts— *Plain Conversation* (*Su Wen*) and *Spiritual Pivot* (*Ling Shu*), each comprising nine volumes, and nine chapters, totaling up to 162 chapters. The author of the book is unknown, and scholars believed that the book summarized the medical ideas before Western Han Dynasty. The book is believed to be the foundation of traditional medical system because it contains complete medical system of Chinese medicine, including yin-yang theory, five elements, life cultivation, syndrome differentiation, visceral manifestation, channels and clinical experience.

Following *Yellow Emperor's Classic of Internal Medicine,* another classic of medicine called *Classic on Difficult Medical Problems* (*Nan Jing*), was given birth to the world before the Eastern Han Dynasty. The book deals mainly with the basic theory of TCM, such as physiology, pathology, diagnosis and treatment of diseases and so on. It supplemented what the *Huangdi's Internal Classic* lacked.

From then on, many medical schools and various classics on medicine were brought into being in succession, each having its own strong points.

Shennong's Classic of Materia Medica (*Shennong Ben Cao Jing*), also known as *Classic of Materia Medica (Ben Cao Jing)* or *Materia Medica* (*Ben Cao*), is the earliest book on materia medica in China, which appeared in the Qin-Han period with its author ship unknown. Not only does it list 365 medicinal items, among which 252 are herbs, 67 are animal medicines, and 46 are mineral medicines. In the book all the medicines are divided into three grades according to their different properties and effects. The book also gives a brief account of pharmacological theories — monarch (*jun*), minister (*chen*), assistant (*zuo*) and guide (*shi*); harmony in seven emotions (*qi qing he he*), four properties of medicinal herbs (*si qi*) and five flavors of medicinal herbs (*wu wei*).

In the Han Dynasty (3rd century AD), Zhang Zhongjing, an outstanding physician, wrote *Treatise on Cold-Attack and Miscellaneous Diseases (Shang Han Za Bing Lun)*, which is divided into two books by later generations, one is entitled *Treatise on Cold Attack* (*Shang Han Lun*), the other *Essentials from the Golden Cabinet (Jin Gui Yao Lüe)*. The book established the principle of syndrome differentiation, there by laying a foundation for the development of clinical medicine.

In the Western Jin Dynasty, Huangfu Mi, a famous physician, compiled *A-B Classic of Acupuncture and Moxibustion (Zhen Jiu Jia Yi Jing)*. The book consists of 12 volumes with 128 chapters, including 349 acupoints. It is the earliest extant work dealing exclusively with acupuncture and moxibustion and one of the most influential works in the history of acupuncture and moxibustion.

The Sui and Tang Dynasties came into their own in feudal economy and culture. In 610 AD, Chao Yuanfang etc. compiled *Treatise on the Causes and Manifestations of Various Diseases (Zhu Bing Yuan Hou Lun)*. The book gave an extensive and minute description of the etiology and symptoms of various diseases. It is the earliest extant classic on etiology and symptoms in China.

In 657 AD, Su Jing together with 20 other scholars, compiled *Newly Revised Materia Medica (Xin Xiu Ben Cao)* , which is the first pharmacopoeia sponsored officially in ancient China, and the earliest pharmacopoeia in the world as well. Sun Simiao (581-682 AD) devoted all his life to writing out two books: *Prescriptions Worth a Thousand Gold Pieces for Emergency (Bei Ji qian Jin Yao Fang)* and *Supplement to Valuable*

Prescriptions (*Qian Jin Yi Fang*). The books deal with general medical theory, materia medica, gynecology and obstetrics, pediatrics, acupuncture and moxibustion, diet, health preservation and prescriptions for various branches of medicine. Sun Simiao was thus honored by later generations as "the king of herbal medicine". Both books are recognized as representative works of medicine in the Tang Dynasty.

In the Song Dynasty, more attention was paid to the education of TCM. The government set up "the Imperial Medical Bureau" for training and bringing up qualified TCM workers.

In 1057 AD, a special organization named "Bureau for Revising Medical Books" was set up in order to proofread and correct the medical books in the past, and to publish them one after another. The books revised have been handed down till now and are still the important classics for China and other countries to study TCM.

In the Jin and Yuan Dynasties, there appeared four medical schools represented by Liu Wansu (1120-1200 AD), Zhang Congzheng (1156-1228 AD), Li Gao (1180-1251 AD) and Zhu Zhenheng (1281-1358 AD). Among them, Liu Wansu believed that "fire and heat" were the main causes of a variety of diseases and that the diseases should be treated with drugs cold and cool in nature. So he was known as "the school of cold and cool" by later generations. Zhang Congzheng believed that all diseases were caused by exogenous pathogenic factors invading the body, and advocated that pathogenic factors should be driven out by methods of diaphoresis, emesis and purgation. So he was known as "the school of purgation". The third school represented by Li Gao, who held that "Internal injuries of the spleen and stomach will bring about various diseases". Therefore, he emphasized that the most important thing, clinically, should be to warm and invigorate the spleen and stomach because the spleen is attributed to the earth in the five elements. So he was regarded as the founder of "the school of reinforcing the earth". And the fourth school was known as "the school of nourishing yin" founded by Zhu Zhenheng. He believed that "Yang is usually redundant, while yin is ever deficient". That is why the body "often has enough yang but not enough yin". So he usually used the method of nourishing yin and purging fire in clinical practice.

Li Shizhen (1518-1593 AD), a famous physician and pharmacologist in the Ming Dynasty, wrote *The Compendium of Materia Medica* (*Ben Cao Gang Mu*). The book consists of 52 volumes with 1,892 medicinal herbs, including over 10,000 prescriptions and 1,000 illustrations of medicinal items. In addition, his book also deals with botany, zoology, mineralogy, physics, astronomy, meteorology, etc. It is really a monumental work in materia medica and a great contribution to the development of pharmacology both in China and all over the world.

During the same period, acupuncture and moxibustion reached their climax. Many literature concerning acupuncture and moxibustion for the ages were summarized and developed.

Since the founding of New China, our government has paid great attention to inheriting and developing the heritage of TCM and materia medica. A series of policies and measures have been taken for developing TCM. In 1986, the National Administrative of Traditional Chinese Medicine was established. In 2013, the Belt and the Road Initiative has ushered in a new era for the fast development of TCM and it's spread to neighboring countries. Never before has TCM been so prosperous as it is today. TCM has experienced many vicissitudes of times but always remains evergreen. There is no doubt that TCM will take its place in medical circles of the world as a completely new medicine.

Questions

(1) Why can TCM exist for such a long time?

(2) What kind of new books on TCM do you expect to see?

(3) What new developments in TCM do you expect?

(4) What limits the development of TCM?

(5) How do you predict the future development of TCM?

V Creative Oral Activity

TCM Heroes in the Pandemic

The past 3 years witnessed a harsh fight between human beings and a virus called coronavirus or COVID-19. During that difficult time, many doctors, including those from the field of TCM worked on the front lines day and night and saved millions of people's lives. Some of them even sacrificed their lives during the so-called "No-smoke" war, like Shi Shuofang, a TCM respiratory disease specialist who was struck by sudden illness during his work in fighting against COVID-19. Shi, also the director of the Jiangsu Province Hospital of Chinese Medicine and professor of Nanjing University of Chinese Medicine, died at 59 in Nanjing.

There are more doctors like Shi, such as Zhang Boli, ChenWei, and Zhang Diying. Prepare a 2-minute speech about your comments on those doctors as well as the lessons that you learn from them.

Chapter Two

TCM vs Western Medicine

Learning Objectives

In this chapter you will learn:

● Differences between Chinese medicine and WM(Western Medicine);

● Different medical treatments for the same disease in two types of medicine;

● Terms related to diseases in Western medicine;

● Different views on Chinese medicine;

● The comparison between TCM and WM in fighting against COVID-19.

I Lead-in Questions

(1) Can you give some examples to illustrate the differences between Chinese and Western medical treatment?

(2) Can you list some advantages of traditional Chinese medicine over Western medicine?

(3) How do you understand the practice "treating headache by needling feet"?

(4) How do you understand the relationship between human health and the natural world?

(5) How is your adaptability to the climatic changes?

(6) What is the effect of geographical and climatic environment on your constitution?

II Useful Expressions

New Words and Phrases

(1) physician /fɪˈzɪʃn/ n. a doctor, especially one who is a specialist in general

medicine and not surgery 医师；内科医生

(2) surgeon /'sɜː dʒən/ *n.* a surgeon is a doctor who is specially trained to perform surgery 外科医生

(3) dredge/dredʒ/ *vt.* to remove mud, stones, etc. from the bottom of a river, canal, etc. using a boat or special machine, to make it deeper or to search for sth. 疏浚；清淤

(4) exuberant /ɪgˈzjuːbərənt/ *adj.* full of energy, excitement and happiness 热情洋溢的；兴高采烈的

(5) abstract /ˈæbstrækt/ *adj.* based on general ideas and not on any particular real person, thing or situation 抽象的

(6) chronic/ˈkrɒnɪk/ *adj.* a chronic illness or disability lasts for a very long time. 慢性的

(7) acute /əˈkjuːt/ *adj.* an acute illness is one that has quickly become severe and dangerous（疾病）急性的

(8) connotation /ˌkɒnəˈteɪʃn/ *n.* an idea suggested by a word in addition to its main meaning 含义；隐含意义

(9) wax/wæks/ *vi.* to become larger, more powerful, etc. 增加；变大

(10) wane/weɪn/*vi.* if something wanes, it becomes gradually weaker or less, often so that it eventually disappears 减弱；减少

(11) pertain to 从属于；适合

(12) static /ˈstætɪk/ *adj.* not moving, changing or developing 静止的；停滞的

(13) substantial /səbˈstænʃl/ *adj.* large and solid; strongly built 大而坚固的；结实的

(14) constituent /kənˈstɪtjuənt/ *n.* one of the parts of sth that combine to form the whole 成分；构成要素

(15) physiology /ˌfɪziˈɒlədʒi/ *n.* the scientific study of the normal functions of living things 生理学

(16) pathology /pəˈθɒlədʒi/ *n.* the scientific study of diseases 病理学

(17) pathological /ˌpæθəˈlɒdʒɪkl/ *adj.* caused by, or connected with, disease or illness 病态的

(18) etiology/ˌiːtɪˈɒlədʒɪ/ *n.* the etiology of a disease or a problem is the study of its causes 病原学

(19) pathogenesis /ˌpæθəˈdʒenɪsɪs/ *n.* (medical 医) the way in which a disease develops 发病机制；病原

(20) holistic /həʊˈlɪstɪk/ *adj.* (informal) considering a whole thing or being to be more than a collection of parts 整体的；全面的

(21) viscera /ˈvɪsərə/ *n.* [pl.] (anatomy 解剖) the large organs inside the body, such as the heart, lungs and stomach 内脏；脏腑

(22) bowels/ˈbaʊəlz/ *n.* your bowels are the tubes in your body through which

digested food passes from your stomach to your anus 肠

 (23) channels /'tʃæn(ə)lz/ *n.* （中医）经脉

 (24) collaterals /kəˈlætərəlz/ *n.* 络脉

 (25) five *zang*-organs 五脏

 (26) six *fu*-organs 六腑

 (27) prevention, treatment and rehabilitation with TCM 中医预防、治疗和康复

 (28) painless acupuncture 无痛针刺

 (29) *tuina* (acupressure) 推拿

 (30) cupping 拔罐

 (31) herbal remedies 草药疗法

 (32) physiological functions 生理功能

 (33) elimination approach 消灭的方法

Sentence Patterns

(1) Traditional Chinese medicine holds that the human body has its own functioning system and people can stay healthy as long as their body system remains balanced.

(2) The effect of TCM therapy for chronic disease is remarkable, while WM is even more outstanding in the treatment of acute disease.

(3) There's still no absolute answer to the question of which form of medicine outperforms the other.

(4) We cannot make simple comparisons between the two types of medicine.

(5) Western medicine considers the human body as a (piece of) machine made up of individual and independent parts.

(6) In western countries, people are beginning to acknowledge the benefits of Chinese medicine.

(7) If you want to produce the best results possible, you can try both TCM and WM at the same time.

(8) Western medicine requires expensive high-tech equipment and extensive chemical manipulation.

(9) The best treatment is to prevent the disease from happening.

(10) TCM encourages people to preserve health while pursuing high moral standards and shouldering social responsibility.

(11) TCM is deeply rooted in the soil of Chinese culture.

(12) TCM reflects the essence and high ethical merits of traditional Chinese culture and continues to enlighten the Chinese nation for the time being.

(13) The unique theoretical system of TCM is the concept of holism and treatment based on syndrome differentiation.

(14) The concept of holism emphasizes the integrity of the human body and the unity between the body and its external environment.

(15) Treatment of a local disease has to take the whole body into consideration.

(16) Drawing yin from yang and drawing yang from yin; treating the right for curing disease on the left, treating the left for curing disease on the right; needling the acupoints on the lower part of the body for the treatment of the disease on the upper part, and needling the acupoints on the upper part of the body for the treatment of the disease on the lower part.

III Model Dialogues

Conversation 1

Jack: People always have confusion when they get sick. I mean, they don't know whether they should choose to see a doctor of Chinese medicine or the one of Western medicine.

Li Ming: Yes, that's because they have no idea about the differences between those medical systems.

Jack: Well, I'd like to hear you talking over it.

Li Ming: The biggest difference between Chinese medicine and Western medicine lies in their theoretical foundations. Chinese medicine is theoretically based on Yin-yang theory, seeking for the balance between yin and yang, so I guess you often hear the saying that "Yin-yang balance ensures human health" .

Jack: Yes, that's true. But there are some other important theories unique to Chinese medicine.

Li Ming: You are right, the theories of Five Elements, *Zang* and *Fu* organs, Channels and Meridians, etc. forms the theoretical basis of Chinese medicine.

Jack: So, what is the theoretical basis of Western medicine?

Li Ming: It is based on anatomy and physiology. The guideline for the treatment in Western medicine is to find out the causes of diseases and eliminate them.

Jack: Wow, that sounds so direct and easy.

Li Ming: But actually, it's not that simple. It is a complicated process involving the diagnosis of doctors combined with examination reports assisted by advanced instruments. When the causes of diseases are confirmed, doctors will give targeted treatment.

Jack: Oh, I see, Chinese medicine attaches more importance to holistic observation over patients, while Western medicine pays more attention to locate the causes of diseases.

Li Ming: You can understand it that way, but it's not right to say that Chinese medicine use comprehensive treatment for all diseases while Western medicine is partial by focusing only on certain local areas of patients. That is the prejudice that some of us hold.

Jack: I understand. Thank you for you explanation.

Li Ming: You're welcome.

Conversation 2

Jack: We have a teamwork project to do: To compare Chinese medicine with Western medicine.

Li Ming: Ok, I think it would be better if we two have a brainstorming before we set down on the presentation, and I will taking notes of our ideas on this notebook.

Jack: Yes. I know Chinese medicine is featured by the concept of holism and treatment based on syndrome differentiation, while Western medicine is characterized by targeting positioning and surgical operations. Take it down.

Li Ming: Good. I've taken it down. Anything else?

Jack: Well, Chinese medicine can address both the symptoms and root of causes for most diseases, but Western medicine may only treat the symptoms.

Li Ming: Well, I think this is arguable. Chinese medicine sometimes puts the treatment of symptoms before that of root causes. For example, if a patient has severe situations like high fever, blood vomiting and coma, doctors will definitely try to stop the situation from getting worse, so in this case symptoms will first be resolved. And Western medicine not only focuses on symptoms, but also the root causes of diseases. For example, for patients who suffer from high fever rising from bacterial infection, doctors will prescribe antibiotics to address the root cause.

Jack: Amazing! I mean your idea is truly impartial and impressive.

Li Ming: Thank you. That's what discussion is for, right? So, go on please. What's the next?

Jack: Chinese medicine takes the Eight Principles as the guideline for diagnosis and the way to recognize the nature of diseases, so doctors of Chinese medicine will decide whether a patient's syndrome belongs to the cold type or heat type, yin type or yang type, etc. However, Western medicine, relies much on experimental data or results.

Li Ming: So we are talking about the differences on diagnosis of diseases between Chinese medicine and Western medicine. I think we'd better include the four diagnostic methods of Chinese medicine in this part.

Jack: Yeah, good idea.

Li Ming: Go on. Any other opinions?

Jack: Hey. Why me again? This is a discussion, rather than an interview. Where is your brain?

Li Ming: Ok, here is one of my ideas. Chinese medicine uses a lot of natural substances, such as herbs, animals and minerals for treatment and all the medicines can be classified into four types according to their properties, like warm, hot, cold and cool. However, Western medicine uses a lot of chemical substances.

Jack: I've taken it down. I think we've gathered enough ideas and we can move to further research before doing the presentation.

Li Ming: Yeah, we worked well with each other.

IV Oral Practice

Situational Dialogues

Situation 1

A madam is suffering from insomnia, and her husband is persuading her to visit a TCM doctor.

Situation 2

Jack is an exchange student studying in Jiangxi, and Lee is a Chinese student studying in Jiangxi University of Chinese Medicine. One day they are arguing with each other over which is better, WM (Western medicine) or TCM.

Situation 3

In 2020, an old lady Madam Wang unfortunately got coronavirus, so she was sent to hospital. The doctor suggested treatment of TCM, but she refused, because she thought it would be too slow to be treated with herbal medicine and it may be useless.

Story Retelling

Cue Words

(1) 葫芦　calabash
(2) 瘟疫　pestilence
(3) 药丸　pill
(4) 恭恭敬敬地　respectfully
(5) 招牌　shop sign; signboard

悬壶济世

我们常称大夫行医的行为是"悬壶济世"。

"壶"就是葫芦。古代没有杯子，人们出门在外时，腰间常悬挂着一个葫芦盛酒水之类，以便路上饮用。喝水用的葫芦怎么会和大夫救死扶伤有关呢？这便要从一个古代传说说起。

相传，东汉时期河南一带闹瘟疫，死了许多人，附近的大夫都无法医治。某日，一位仙风道骨的老者来到这里，开始普济患病的百姓，他看病的方式很奇特。老翁在门前挂了一个葫芦，凡是有人求医，他就从葫芦里取出一粒药丸，让患者用水冲服。吃药的人没过多久便一个个痊愈了，瘟疫也随之消散了。

当时，有一个叫费长房的年轻人断定这位老翁绝非等闲之辈，便想跟随他学医，于是他买了酒肉，恭恭敬敬地拜见这位老翁。老翁见费长房诚心求学，便收他为徒，领他一同进入了那个取药的葫芦中，在葫芦里教授他治病的本领。

从此，费长房也能医百病，驱瘟疫，令人起死回生，成为一代名医。费长房为了纪念他的师父，行医时总是在腰间系上一个葫芦，把药物储存在里边。这件事广为流传，因此大夫们在行医时，便也用葫芦当招牌，以表示自己医术高超，老百姓们也因此把葫芦当作大夫的标记。

如今，虽然在中医大夫门前"悬壶"的习惯已经没有了，但"悬壶济世"这一说法却一直沿用至今。其实，在这个成语中，"悬壶"只是形式，"济世"才是根本，无论形式如何变，葫芦也好，罐子也罢，最重要的是那颗救人于水火的济世仁爱之心。

Group Task

As the COVID-19 pandemic continues to spread across the world, we understand that many countries are under stress due to its blow to the global economy and social order. COVID-19 knows no borders and it is important for us to share the experience and learn the effective measures taken in different countries. Over the past five months, China has been facing a big challenge against COVID-19 pandemic while it has been controlled pretty well so far. In response to the coronavirus in China, TCM has made great contributions and the results are surprisingly good. TCM treatment has a good effect on improving the overall condition of patients, relieving symptoms and shortening the course of the disease. Also, it has a wide and deep range of participation and gets a large amount of attention. The treatment of integrating Chinese and Western medicine has played a key role in China's COVID-19 prevention and control and made significant contributions to China's initial victory against the pandemic.

Oral Task

Work with your teammates and gather information about TCM's contribution to resist

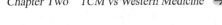

and cure infectious diseases in human history. Please prepare a PowerPoint and display it in class.

Reading and Question Answering

Contrast Between TCM and Western Medicine Technology

There are many differences between Chinese medicine and Western medicine. For example, TCM focuses on people in terms of treating diseases, while Western medicine targets at diseases. Two examples are discussed in this article: first, pulse measurement in Western medicine and pulse-taking in TCM; Second, the injection needles and TCM acupuncture.

(1) Pulse measurement and pulse-taking

In Western medicine, doctors observe the patients' heart beat by measuring the pulse, or they use medical instrument to gather data about heart beat, such as sphygmomanometer, which can not only measure the pulse but also blood pressure. The use of medical instruments in Western medicine helps doctors to better understand the conditions of a patient's health and diseases. Compared with pulse diagnosis in Western medicine, TCM doctors attach importance to the flow of *qi* and blood rather than heart beat. It is an important idea in Chinese medicine that humans correspond with the natural world, so the pulse manifestation, to some extent, reflects the interaction between humans and natural environment.

As for pulse-taking, it is one of the four diagnostic methods widely used in Chinese medicine. There are three pulse positions for pulse taking, namely *Cun, Guan* and *Chi*. When the doctor gently puts his finger on the *"Cun"* position of the patient's right wrist, he can tell the condition of the large intestine, while the condition of the stomach can be detected by the adjacent fingers. This medical diagnostic skill relies much on the physician's personal medical experience, which is different from health examination in Western medicine.

(2) Needles in Western medicine and TCM

In Western medicine, a needle is a hollow sharp tube through which drugs can be injected to a patient's body. How the needle is perfectly inserted into the blood vessel depends on a nurse's knowledge of anatomy as well as practical skills.

The acupuncture needle used in Chinese medicine is usually silver and solid. The needles are used to regulate *qi* flowing in channels by stimulating certain acupoints. TCM often uses the combination of the two methods—acupuncture and moxibustion. The needling methods of Chinese acupuncture are complicated, and needles in TCM can be used in various ways to achieve different healing purposes, considering factors like the depth of acupoints, the time for retaining the needle and pulling it out, and whether moxibustion therapy should be combined.

Questions

(1) What are the differences between pulse measurement in Western medicine and pulse taking in TCM?

(2) Can you summarize the differences between TCM and WM mentioned in the article? Are there any other differences between them? (Search for more information online)

V Creative Oral Activity

TCM Cannot Flourish Without Ancient Wisdom

Traditional Chinese medicine is a medical system developed through thousands of years of practice. Although informed by modern medicine, TCM is built on the foundation of more than 2,500 years of Chinese medical practice that includes herbal medicines, exercise, massage, acupuncture and dietary therapy.

As a traditional medical system, TCM has made significant contributions to the health and prosperity of Chinese people, and during different Chinese dynasties, medical experts have summed up their valuable experience of medicine regimes and treatment in a series of books.

When the country was struggling to control the novel coronavirus, TCM proved to be effective as a therapy. According to the State Council Information Office, more than 90 percent of the COVID-19 patients in China have received TCM treatment and 90 percent of those have benefited from it. Practice shows that TCM has advantages in terms of pandemic control and prevention. It can effectively prevent infection, cure mild symptoms before they develop into serious cases, and shorten the time of recovery.

As President Xi Jinping said, one bright spot of China's experience in the fight against the pandemic is the integration of TCM and Western medicine, which is another example of TCM facilitating innovative practices in the use of modern medicine.

As two branches of medical science, TCM and Western medicine have a common goal: curing diseases. Yet they have differences in theory, treatment and curative effects. Influenced by traditional Chinese philosophy, TCM is a holistic medical system. It focuses on analyzing an individual's functional identities (which regulate digestion, breathing, blood circulation), and views overall health as the harmonious interaction between these identities and the outside world. TCM diagnosis aims to trace the symptoms to the patterns of an underlying disharmony by, for example, measuring the pulse, checking the tongue and eyes, and analyzing the eating and sleeping habits of an individual.

By contrast, Western medicine uses clinical diagnosis and medical tests (for instance, blood tests) to prescribe pharmaceutical drugs and other therapeutics to cure a disease. Although Western medicine is more objective than TCM, it is less concerned about the human body as a whole as it focuses on the symptoms to treat a disease.

Despite their differences, TCM and Western medicine have their respective advantages and therefore can complement one another. So there is no reason to belittle TCM in comparison with Western medicine, though TCM has some limitations despite its continued development through the centuries.

TCM's vitality comes from a wealth of clinical experiences that have proved effective in practice. TCM is holistic in nature, and its further development depends on its historical legacy, adopting modern diagnosis methods and developing innovate ways to treat diseases. To modernize TCM, practitioners have to make full use of modern science and promote interdisciplinary cooperation.

Yet TCM is deeply influenced by ancient philosophy and the cosmological notion of yin and yang. So to adapt to modern practices, TCM has to follow Western rules of medical science and pharmaceutical drugs, including practicing evidence-based treatment and standardization of diagnosis and prognosis methods, while reducing the role of traditional Chinese culture.

But by focusing excessively on quantitative research and evidence-based medical science, and neglecting qualitative study and abstract thought, TCM will veer away from the cultural soil on which it has flourished for thousands of years. Evidence-based medical science cannot interpret the wisdom of TCM, especially in terms of its curative effect on chronic diseases and infections — because it is difficult for modern science to explain its treatment process.

Without the nutrients from traditional Chinese philosophy and culture, it will be difficult for TCM to develop in the future. Thus, only by following traditional Chinese culture and philosophy can we promote the development of TCM in the future.

Questions

(1) What are the differences between Chinese and Western medicine according to the article?

(2) Jiangxi has always been labeled as a powerful province for its TCM industries and cultural deposits, how can you introduce Jiangxi from the perspective of TCM?

(3) What can we do to promote the internationalization of TCM?

Chapter Three

Yin-yang Theory

Learning Objectives

In this chapter you will learn:

● How to introduce the concept of yin and yang and their relationships in English;

● How to apply yin-yang theory in physiology, pathology and diagnosis;

● A series of conversational skills and practice related with the topic of yin and yang.

I Lead-in Questions

(1) What is the meaning of yin and yang in your opinion?

(2) Can you name some examples to represent yin and yang?

(3) What are the relations between yin and yang?

(4) What is the value of yin and yang considering human health?

II Useful Expressions

New Words and Phrases

(1) convert /kənˈvɜːt/ *vt.* change the nature, purpose, or function of something 使转变

(2) alternation /ˌɔːltəˈneɪʃn/ *n.* successive change from one thing or state to another and back again 交替，轮流

(3) exhaustion /ɪgˈzɔːstʃən/ *n.* the act of exhausting something entirely *n.* 枯竭；耗尽

(4) physiology /ˌfɪziˈɒlədʒi/ *n.* the branch of the biological sciences dealing with the functioning of organisms 生理学

(5) organ /ˈɔːgən/ *n.* a fully differentiated structural and functional unit in an animal

that is specialized for some particular function 器官

(6) tissue /ˈtɪʃuː/ *n.* part of an organism consisting of an aggregate of cells having a similar structure and function 组织

(7) fluid /ˈfluːɪd/ *n.* a continuous amorphous substance that tends to flow 液体

(8) deficiency /dɪˈfɪʃnsi/ *n.* lack of an adequate quantity or number 缺乏

(9) nourish /ˈnʌrɪʃ/ *v.* provide with nourishment 滋养

(10) marrow /ˈmærəʊ/ *n.* the fatty network of connective tissue that fills the cavities of bones 髓，骨髓

(11) antibiotic /ˌæntibaɪˈɒtɪk/ *adj.* of or relating to antibiotic drugs 抗菌的

(12) harmony /ˈhɑːməni/ *n.* a harmonious state of things in general and of their properties (as of colors and sounds); congruity of parts with one another and with the wholeness 和谐

(13) pathological /ˌpæθəˈlɒdʒɪkl/ *adj.* caused by or altered by or manifesting disease or pathology 病理学的；病态的

(14) diagnosis /ˌdaɪəgˈnəʊsɪs/ *n.* identifying the nature or cause of some phenomenon 诊断

(15) complementary /ˌkɒmplɪˈmentri/ *adj.* acting as or providing a complement (something that completes the whole) 补足的

(16) essence /ˈesns/ *n.* that which makes a thing what it is; most important or indispensable quality of sth. （中医上指）精气；精

(17) descend /dɪˈsend/ *vi.* move downward and lower, but not necessarily all the way. 下降

(18) metabolism /məˈtæbəlɪzəm/ *n.* the organic processes (in a cell or organism) that are necessary for life 新陈代谢

(19) wax /wæks/ *vi.* increase in phase 增大

(20) wane /weɪn/ *vi.* grow smaller 衰落；变小

(21) epilepsy /ˈepɪlepsi/ *n.* a disorder of the nervous system that causes a person to become unconscious suddenly, often with violent movements of the body 癫痫；羊痫风

(22) histological /histəˈlɒdʒikəl/ *adj.* 组织学的

(23) encompass /ɪnˈkʌmpəs/ *vt.* to include a large number or range of things 包含

(24) vibrant /ˈvaɪbrənt/ *adj.* full of life and energy 充满生机的

Sentence Patterns

● How to introduce the idea of harmony and the idea of yin and yang

(1) Yin and yang is one of the most fundamental concepts in traditional Chinese medicine.

(2) The concept of yin and yang is essentially simple, yet its influence on Chinese

culture has been extensive.

(3) The yin and yang are two opposite principles in nature.

(4) Yin and yang can be regarded as complementary forces.

(5) The yin and yang are two opposite principles in nature. Yin is associated with the negative aspects and it symbolizes feminine character. Yang is associated with positive qualities and it symbolizes the character of male.

(6) The balance between yin and yang is important in Chinese culture. Chinese believe that the idea of yin and yang exist in every aspect of life, such as female and male, cold and hot, dark and bright, moon and sun, sadness and happiness, etc.

(7) The Chinese symbol for yin is the shaded side of a hill. It signifies femininity, coolness, dampness, and darkness. In contrast, yang is the sunny side of the hill. It signifies masculinity, warmth, dryness, and light.

(8) The early connotations of yin and yang were quite simple, the side facing the sun being yang and the reverse side being yin.

(9) As observation of yin and yang deepened, ancient Chinese realized that everything in the universe has two opposite aspects whose interactions promoted development and change.

(10) The best example to show the contradiction between yin and yang is the relation between water and fire as described in *Su Wen* that "Water and fire are the symbols of yin and yang."

(11) Yin and yang oppose each other. The opposition between yin and yang means that all things or phenomena in the natural world have two opposite aspects known as yin and yang, such as heaven and earth, motion and quiescence, ascending and descending, exiting and entering, day and night, heat and cold, etc.

(12) Yin and yang depend on each other. Without yin there would be no yang, and vice versa. When the interdependent relationships between substances, between functions as well as between substances and functions get abnormal, life activities will be broken, thus bringing about dissociation of yin and yang, depletion of essence, and even an end of life.

(13) Yin and yang wane and wax between each other. yin and yang coexist in a dynamic equilibrium in which one waxes while the other wanes. In other words, waning of yin will lead to waxing of yang and vice versa.

(14) Yin and yang transform between each other. Under given conditions, either yin or yang may transform into its counterpart.

(15) It is said in *Su Wen* that "Extreme yin turns into yang, and extreme yang turns into yin" and "Extreme cold brings on heat, and extreme heat brings on cold".

(16) After Zou Yan put forward the "Five Virtues" theory, yin and yang and the five

elements were also used in politics, such as deducing the replacement of dynasties, ghosts and gods, misfortunes and blessings, and predicting, etc.

(17) The theory of yin and yang and five elements is widely used in the field of agricultural production and medicine.

(18) Conventional fields of western nutrition classify food in terms of its chemical composition, including the calories, carbohydrates, proteins, fats, and other nutrients that it contains. TCM focuses on the energy properties of food. According to TCM, a balance of "cool" and "hot" foods, or yin and yang foods, is essential to good health.

(19) To achieve harmony of your body, mind, and *qi*, it is important to eat yin-yang-balanced foods.

(20) Yin foods are believed to be cool and thought to moisten your body. Yang foods are believed to be warm and drying.

(21) "Cool" or yin foods are generally low in calories and high in potassium. They're recommended in hot weather. "Hot" or yang foods tend to be higher in calories and sodium. They're recommended in colder months to help warm your body.

(22) Common yin foods include:

➢ soy products, such as tofu and soybean sprouts;
➢ certain meats, such as crab and duck;
➢ fruit, such as watermelon and star fruit;
➢ vegetables, such as watercress, cucumbers, carrots, and cabbage;
➢ cold drinks and water.

Common yang foods include:

➢ foods that are high in fat, protein, calories, and sodium;
➢ certain meats, such as chicken, pork, and beef;
➢ warm spices, such as cinnamon, nutmeg, and ginger;
➢ eggs, glutinous rice, sesame oil, bamboo, and mushrooms;
➢ alcoholic beverages.

(23) In human bodies, the back is yang and the abdomen is yin. The six *fu*-organs are yang and the five *zang*-organs are yin. Keeping balance of yin and yang will lead to a healthy and vibrant life.

● How to apply yin-yang theory in physiology, pathology and diagnosis

(1) The theory of yin and yang serves to explain the organic structure, physiological function and pathological changes of the human body, and in addition, guides clinical diagnosis and treatment.

(2) Physiologically, the theory of yin and yang holds that the normal life activities of the human body result from the coordination between yin and yang in a unity of opposites.

(3) Take the relationship between the function and substance for example, the

function pertains to yang while substance to yin.

(4) Without functional activities, the metabolism of the substance will be impossible to be carried out; without necessary substance, the functional activities will have no way to be performed.

(5) Pathologically, TCM considers that the imbalance between yin and yang is one of the basic pathogenesis of disease.

(6) The course of a disease is actually the process of the struggle between the healthy *qi* and pathogenic factors that consequently leads to relative predominance and decline of yin and yang in the organism.

(7) Heat syndrome caused by preponderance of yang, for example, belongs to excess heat syndrome. It should be treated with herbs cold in nature in order to inhibit predominant yang so as to cool the heat.

(8) As to the flavor of the herbs, those that are sour, bitter and salty in taste belong to yin and those that are acrid, sweet and bland in taste pertain to yang.

(9) When the balance between yin and yang in the body is destroyed, there can be a series of pathological changes, called "yin and yang disharmony" in TCM.

III Model Dialogues

Conversation 1

Jack: Hi, Li. I am truly interested in yin-yang theory from Chinese medicine, but it's so hard to understand.

Li Ming: Tell me what confuses you, and I'd like to see if I can answer some of your questions.

Jack: Well, it is believed in Chinese medicine that everything in the universe can be classified into either the yin type or the yang type, which is too abstract for me to understand.

Li Ming: I know it's not easy to accept the concept of yin and yang. In ancient times, people held that the source and original state of the universe was "qi" which produced two poles known as "yin" and "yang". Since everything in the universe is produced during the motion and interaction of qi, so it is natural that everything possesses the properties of yin or yang.

Jack: Oh, I see. No wonder everything in the universe has its opposite side, such as the day and the night, water and fire, upper and lower, cold and hot, women and men, etc.

Li Ming: Yes, you are right.

Jack: What on earth is the meaning of yin and yang in Chinese culture?

Li Ming: The original meaning of yin and yang is simple and concrete. The mountain slope facing the sun refers to yang, while the side where sunlight could not reach is called yin.

Jack: So yang means "sunshine" while yin means "shadow".

Li Ming: Yes, you can understand it that way.

Jack: Another thing that troubles me is how to decide the nature of something in terms of yin-yang theory.

Li Ming: Yes, sometimes the properties of things expressed by yin-yang theory is truly abstract. So ancient Chinese use specific examples like water and fire to signify the nature of yin and yang respectively.

Jack: That's easy to understand. There is such an obvious contrast between water and fire. Fire is warm, bright and up-flaming, while water is cold, dim, peaceful and downward flowing. What about something like a TABLE? How do I know whether it pertains to yin or yang?

Li Ming: Good question. There is not a definite answer to your question, because you get different answers when you see the table from different aspects.

Jack: I don't see...

Li Ming: Well, the bottom of the table pertains to yin, while the top of it pertains to yang. If the table is red, it pertains to yang, while a blue table pertains to yin. If it is a new table, it pertains to yang, while an old table yin. It varies.

Jack: Oh, I see. It's dynamic. Thank you for your explanation.

Conversation 2

Jack: I was told that anything with the properties of being warm, bright, active, rising and dispersing pertains to yang, while the things having the properties of being cold, dim, static, descending and astringing pertain to yin.

Li Ming: Wow, it seems you know quite a lot about yin-yang theory in Chinese medicine.

Jack: You are flattering me. I really don't know how to apply that theory into my life.

Li Ming: Well, it would help us a lot if we can adhere to yin-yang theory. Take food for example, there are yin-type and yang-type food. And if we eat in the right way, we will enjoy good health.

Jack: This is surely something new to me. Can you give me some examples of food belonging to different types?

Li Ming: Well, that's easy. Usually fruits, vegetables and seaweeds pertain to yin, while animal meat, fish and shellfish pertain to yang. As to the flavors of food, sour food generally pertains to yin, whereas salty food pertains to yang.

Jack: Oh, I see. So fruits like watermelon, pear and durian are yin by nature, right?

Li Ming: Not exactly, there are exceptions. Durian, due to its high calories and sugar, belongs to the yang type.

Jack: Then, how can I correctly incorporate the yin-yang theory into my daily diet?

Li Ming: That depends on your constitution. I mean you should adjust your diet to suit your physiological condition.

Jack: I don't see what you mean. How do I know what type of constitution I belong to?

Li Ming: Well, you need to seek for the professional suggestions from doctors of Chinese medicine. Some people may easily get internal heat, so they should consume some yin-type food to clear away the excessive heat in their body, while those belonging to the yin-deficient constitution should try to eat some yang-type food to supplement the energy in their body.

Jack: That sounds reasonable. And it seems that I still have a lot to learn in Chinese medicine. Thank you, Li.

Li Ming: Not at all.

IV Oral Practice

Situational Dialogues

Situation 1

Lucy is an exchange student from the USA. She has been living in China for 5 years and she noticed that Chinese people attach great importance to the balance of yin and yang, not only in the field of health conservation, but also in other aspects, such as *fengshui*, four seasons, family relationship and so on. You are a student majoring in TCM and you start up a conversation with Lucy.

Situation 2

Jack is learning traditional Chinese medicine in Beijing University of Chinese medicine. Recently, he was puzzled by some expressions he read from *Huangdi's Internal Classic*, such as "extreme cold generates heat", "extreme heat generates cold", "excessive yin turns into yang", and "excessive yang turns into yin". You hold a discussion with Jack in TCM class.

Story Retelling

Cue Words

(1) 乐极生悲　extreme joy begets sorrow
(2) 不理朝政　ignore government affairs
(3) 沉溺于　indulge in
(4) 侵扰　invade and harass
(5) 齐威王　The king of *qi*
(6) 醉酒的　get drunk
(7) 斛是中国古代量器名，也是容量单位。古代常用容量单位由小到大有升、斗、（石）、釜、钟，五斗为一斛，十斗为一石。淳于髡（kūn）说的“我喝一斗也醉，喝一石也醉”可以意译为：I may get drunk if I drink either a cup or a pot.
(8) 极致　extremes

乐极生悲的典故

战国时期，齐威王不理朝政，经常通宵沉溺在酒色中，诸侯趁机侵扰，国家处于危亡之际。大臣们谁也不敢规劝，只是干着急。齐国有个叫淳于髡的人，他说话诙谐善辩，喜欢用隐语、微言齐讽谏威王的过失。

有一次，楚国大规模发兵侵犯齐国，齐威王急忙派自己信任的大臣淳于髡去赵国求救。淳于髡最终不负齐威王的重托，到赵国请来了十万大军，成功吓退了楚军。齐威王非常高兴，立刻摆设酒宴请淳于髡喝酒庆贺。齐威王兴奋地问淳于髡：“先生，你要喝多少酒才会醉？”淳于髡看这架势，知道齐威王又要彻夜喝酒，一醉方休了。他想了想回答道：“我喝一斗酒也醉，喝一石酒也醉。”

齐威王觉得淳于髡的话很奇怪，问道：“你淳于髡到底是一斗的量还是一石的量呢？”淳于髡回答说：“我听说喝酒到了极致，就会酒醉从而乱了礼节；人一旦快乐到了极点，就可能会发生让人悲伤的事情了。任何事情都是一样的，如果超过一个限度，就会走向反面。”

齐威王知道淳于髡是在委婉地规劝他，这一席话也让自己心服口服，他当即表示接受淳于髡的劝告，从今以后不会再彻夜饮酒作乐，改掉这个恶习。如此，淳于髡救了齐威王和齐国。“乐极生悲”这一成语便是从这个故事中得来，形容高兴到极点时，就会发生使人悲伤的事情。

Group Task

The theory of yin and yang is a way to look at the universe as well as a method used by the ancient Chinese to understand and explain nature. Work in groups to find some concrete examples which reflect duality in daily life to illustrate the theory of yin and yang. Please present your findings in PPT.

Reading and Question Answering

When it comes to Japan's representative culture, most people may immediately think of things such as anime, kimonos or sushi. Recently, however, a different part of traditional Japanese culture-Onmyodo, or the *Way of Yin Yang*-has been gaining ground in China due to a new popular video game.

Onmyoji (Master of *Yin* and *Yang*) is a mobile roleplaying game produced by Netease Inc., NTES, a Chinese game company, that takes place in Japan during the Heian Period (794-1192). The game was officially released on June 1, 2016 for Android users and was later brought to iPhones three months later.

The game became a huge hit in the Chinese, Japanese and South Korean markets almost immediately after it debuted. According to Netease, the game attracted more than 10 million daily active users within its first 50 days.

"I have to say, the art style and special effects during combat are really well done, as is the story and music," netizen Reality winner/Dream loser, wrote on Zhihu, a Chinese question and answer platform concerning his impressions about the game.

The initial inspiration for this game can be traced back to *The Tale of Genji*, a novel written by Murasaki Shikibu (973-1025), a famous female writer from the Heian Period. The story, however, comes from the novel *Onmyoji,* a fantasy work by Japanese writer Yumemakura Baku that depicts extraordinary stories involving humans and ghosts.

"One of the most attractive points for the game Onmyoji is that it uses a lot of Japanese elements but is produced by Chinese, which puts to rest the argument that Chinese cannot produce things with a Japanese style well," netizen Seanli posted on Chinese game website Game Dog.

A deeper look at Onmyoji reveals that it is not just imitating a Japanese style game, but is actually an excellent combination of both Chinese and Japanese elements.

Though the concept of Yin and Yang is an ingrained part of Japanese culture, it actually originates from China. At their most basic, Yang means facing the sun, while Yin means having one's back to the sun. Ancient Chinese expanded the basic meaning of these two contrary concepts into a philosophy in which the natural order of the universe is explained in terms of interconnected duality such as male and female, positive and negative and so on. The beginnings of Yin Yang theory can be traced to a time when China was made up of numerous independent tribal cultures. It continued to evolve and change over the centuries, reaching its full development as a complicated theory during the late Han Dynasty (206BC-AD220).

Inheriting the concept of Yin Yang from China, Japan further extended it to astronomy, economics, politics and divination. As more Japanese elements were introduced, it became more and more popular. In fact, Onmyoji (Lit: Yin Yang master) eventually became an official government position that had an important role when it came to calendar science and even official policy decisions.

"It is easy to see that this Chinese game company has combined two cultures by producing a Japanese-styled game themed after Yin and Yang. It reminds me of the Tang Dynasty (618-907), a time when Japanese came to China to study the Tang's advanced culture and bring it back to Japan. Later, we imported the Japanese tea ceremony and the art of flower arrangement," Seanli wrote.

"This fusion of cultures makes the world a better place."

Questions

(1) In which aspect is yin-yang theory used?
(2) Why can yin-yang theory win the favor from other countries?

V Creative Oral Activity

For many people, the theory of yin and yang is regarded as a thinking mode for Chinese ancients and some believe it is outdated. Although the yin-yang theory has a history of thousands of years, it is still applied in modern society, which is very helpful to guide our living habits, explain and deal with many life problems. This is also fully in line with our current spirit of promoting traditional culture, so the yin-yang theory is indeed the essence of our traditional culture. After learning this chapter, can you share your plan to use yin-yang theory to improve your health and life?

Chapter Four

Five Elements
....

Learning Objectives

In this chapter you will learn:

● How to introduce the theory of five elements;

● How to apply the five elements in diagnosis and treatment;

● A series of conversational expressions on the given topics.

I Lead-in Questions

(1) What are the five elements in TCM?

(2) What are the features of "wood" in nature and what about the "wood" in five elements?

(3) What are the relationships among those five elements?

II Useful Expressions

New Words and Phrases

(1) transform /træns'fɔːm/ *vt.* change or alter in form, appearance, or nature 转换

(2) lung /lʌŋ/ *n.* either of two sack-like respiratory organs in the chest serving for breathing 肺

(3) gallbladder /ˈgɔːl,blædə/ *n.* a muscular sac attached to the liver that secretes bile and stores it until needed for digestion 胆囊

(4) intestine /ɪnˈtestɪn/ *n.* the part of the alimentary canal between the stomach and the anus 肠

(5) kidney /ˈkɪdni/ *n.* either of two bean-shaped excretory organs that filter wastes (especially urea) from the blood and excrete them and water in urine 肾脏

(6) phlegm /flem/ *n.* the thick substance that forms in the nose and throat, especially when you have a cold 痰

(7) generative /ˈdʒenərətɪv/ *adj.* producing new life or offspring 生殖的

(8) reinforce /ˌriːɪnˈfɔːs/ *vt.* to make sth. stronger 加强；加固

(9) adverse /ˈædvɜːs/ *adj.* contrary to your interests or welfare 不利的

(10) dysfunction /dɪsˈfʌŋkʃn/ *n.* (medicine) any disturbance in the function of an organ or body part 功能紊乱

(11) retention /rɪˈtenʃn/ *n.* the act of retaining something 滞留

(12) peripheral /pəˈrɪfərəl/ *a.* of or in a periphery 周围的；边缘的

(13) interact /ˌɪntərˈækt/ *v.* to have an effect on each other or something else by being or working close together 互相作用；互相影响

(14) cereal /ˈsɪəriəl/ *n.* any kind of grain 谷物

(15) nutrient /ˈnjuːtriənt/ *n.* (a chemical or food) providing for life and growth 养分；营养物

(16) synthesize /ˈsɪnθəsaɪz/ *v.* to make up or produce by combining parts 综合

(17) ascension /əˈsenʃn/ *n.* (formal) the act of moving up or of reaching a high position 上升

(18) referral /rɪˈfɜːrəl/ *n.* 转诊的病人

(19) dysfunction /dɪsˈfʌŋkʃən/ *n.* if someone has a physical dysfunction, part of their body is not working properly 机能障碍；功能不良

(20) mass /mæs/ *n.* a small, hard swelling that has been caused by an injury or an illness 肿块

(21) cyst /sɪst/ *n.* a cyst is a growth containing liquid that appears inside your body or under your skin 囊肿

(22) gland /ɡlænd/ *n.* a gland is an organ in the body which produces chemical substances for the body to use or get rid of 腺

(23) brittle /ˈbrɪtəl/ *adj.* an object or substance that is hard but easily broken 硬脆易碎的

(24) elicit /ɪˈlɪsɪt/ *vt.* if you elicit a response or a reaction, you do or say something that makes other people respond or react 引起（反应）

(25) engender /ɪnˈdʒendə(r)/ *vi.* (formal) to make a feeling or situation exist 产生；引起

(26) restrain /rɪˈstreɪn/ *vt.* keep under control; keep in check 抑制；控制

(27) excess /ɪkˈses/ *n.* a quantity much larger than is needed 过度；过量

(28) overwhelm /əʊvəˈwelm/ *vt.* one element in the five elements excessively restrains another element 相乘

(29) subjugate /ˈsʌbdʒuɡeɪt/ *v.* defeating and making obedient 征服，（中医指）相乘

(30) rebellion /rɪˈbeljən/ *n.* an abnormal state in which one element in the five

elements reversely restrain and bullies another element 相侮

(31) wood, fire, earth, metal and water 木、火、土、金、水

(32) wood generates/ promotes fire 木生火

(33) wood restricts/ restrains earth 木克土

(34) fire subjugates/ over-restrains metal 火乘金

(35) metal counter-restricts/ rebels fire 金侮火

Sentence Patterns

How to introduce the theory of five elements

(1) The five elements refer to wood, fire, earth, metal and water as well as their motion and changes in the natural world.

(2) Developed by *Zou Yan* (350-270 BC), during the Warring States period (475-221 BC), five-element theory became popular and was applied to medicine.

(3) The theory of the five elements holds that all phenomena in the universe correspond in nature either to wood, fire, earth, metal or water, and that these elements are in a state of constant motion and change.

(4) Wood is characterized by growing freely and peripherally. So anything with the functions of growing and developing freely is attributed to the category of wood.

(5) Fire is characterized by flaming up. Thereby anything with the functions of warming and rising is attributed to the category of fire.

(6) Earth is characterized by cultivation and reaping. So anything with the functions of generating, transforming, supporting and receiving is attributed to the category of earth.

(7) Metal is characterized by change. Hence anything with the functions of purifying, descending and astringing is attributed to the category of metal.

(8) Water is characterized by moistening and downward flowing. Therefore, anything with the functions of cooling, moistening and moving downward is attributed to the category of water.

(9) The relationship of the five elements can be summarized as generation, restriction, subjugation, and counter-restriction, and mutual interaction between mother-element and child-element.

(10) The five-element theory is the foundation of Chinese disciplines such as *fengshui*, the martial arts and the *I Ching(Book of Changes)*.

How to apply the five elements in diagnosis and treatment

(11) Each of the internal organs, according to the theory of five elements, pertains to

one of the five elements.

(12) The liver prefers to grow freely and dislikes depression, so it pertains to wood.

(13) The heart pumps blood to warm the body, thereby it pertains to fire.

(14) The spleen is responsible for transforming and transporting cereal nutrients to all parts of the body, thus it pertains to earth.

(15) The lung is marked by the functions of purification and descending, for that reason it pertains to metal.

(16) The kidney is in charge of storing essence and governing water, therefore it pertains to water.

(17) The relationships of the five elements play an important role in maintaining a balanced lifestyle.

(18) During the spring season, which belongs to the wood element, we should avoid excessive anger in order to stay healthy.

(19) The kidney corresponds to water in five-element theory. Just as water supports the growth and development of plants, the kidney supports the birth, development and maturation of humans.

(20) The liver is related with the wood element and controls the flow of *qi*. If a person is excessively angry, the liver will be adversely affected.

III Model Dialogues

Conversation 1

Jack: Hi, Li Ming. You know what. Yesterday I met a real master in Chinese medicine. He is a real expert on five elements.

Li Ming: Really? How do you know it?

Jack: Well, the moment I stepped into his clinic, I was impressed and stunned by the decoration in it. There was a large wooden table in the east side of clinic, a stove in the south, a clock hanging on the west wall, a water vat in the north and a large flower pot containing yellow mud in the middle.

Li Ming: Wow, the decoration is truly interesting, and seems to be a good demonstration of five-element theory, but I would say something different from what you think.

Jack: What do you mean?

Li Ming: I mean the doctor of Chinese medicine you saw yesterday may not be a real TCM master. He may not grasp the real meaning of five elements, so it is totally a showing-off to decorate his clinic like that.

Jack: I cannot see what you mean. As I know, five elements are related with five directions and there seems to be nothing wrong with the decoration.

Li Ming: Yes, the part of relation between five elements with five direction is right. But maybe you have misunderstandings on five elements.

Jack: I'd like to listen to your interpretation.

Li Ming: Well, five elements in Chinese medicine, such as wood, fire, earth, metal and water, are different from the five kinds of tangible substances we see in the natural world. Actually, they refer to five kinds of properties. Take water for example, it is cold and cool, soft and nourishing, and it has the features of flowing downwards and supplementing the growth of wood. So anything sharing the similar features like water falls into water.

Jack: Oh, I suddenly realize that this is the typical thinking mode possessed by Chinese. That is, to use concrete examples to signify an obvious feature or a kind of property.

Li Ming: Yes, you are right. Just like water is chosen to represent yin, and fire yang.

Jack: In this sense, it is truly misleading that the doctor of the clinic uses five kinds of substances to represent five elements in Chinese medicine.

Li Ming: Or, maybe you get the doctor wrong. He just thought it was beautiful to decorate his clinic like that. It was you who speculated the connection between five elements and the decoration.

Conversation 2

Jack: I know the number five is a special figure in traditional Chinese medicine, and there are many important terms containing the number five, such as five sounds, five flavors, five colors, etc.

Li Ming: Yes, you are right, and nearly all of them are related with five elements. For example, the five internal organs are corresponding to five elements.

Jack: I know it. Liver corresponds to wood, heart to fire, spleen to earth, lungs to metal and kidney to water.

Li Ming: I can see that you're serious about the course of Chinese medicine.

Jack: Yes, I have strong interest in this course from which I learn the collective wisdom of ancient Chinese, but I have to say I still have a lot of puzzlement on five elements. For example, what is on earth the use of this abstract theory in medical practice?

Li Ming: Well, the theory of five elements is one of the basic theories in Chinese medicine, and it is vitally important for guiding the clinical practice in Chinese medicine. For example, it helps to explain the physiological functions of the five *zang*-organs and their relationships.

Jack: I don't see what you mean.

Li Ming: Well, just like the relationships among five elements, there are also the relations of generation, restriction, subjugation and counter-restriction among five *zang*-organs. For example, the blood stored in the liver helps to nourish the heart spirit, so the liver can promote the functions of the heart. Likewise, heart spirit can help regulate the transporting and transforming functions of the spleen.

Jack: Oh, I see. This shows that the five *zang*-organs can support each other. What about the reflection of restriction and counter-restriction?

Li Ming: Under pathological conditions, disorders of one organ may be transmitted to another, which are generally caused by the relations of restriction and counter-restriction. For example, if liver-*qi* invades the spleen, it will affect the functions of the spleen. Another example is that if the liver fire is too exuberant, it will invade the lungs, leading to the dysfunctions of the lungs.

Jack: Thank you for your explanation. I understand more about the theory of five elements.

Li Ming: You're welcome.

IV Oral Practice

Situational Dialogues

Work in teams and make up dialogues based on the following situations.

Situation 1

Both you and Xiao Zhang are students majoring in TCM and you are good friends. Today, you have learnt knowledge of five elements in TCM. Xiao Zhang is sick, so he/she failed to attend the class, and you help him/her with today's class.

Situation 2

Xiao Zhang is a student majoring in Chinese medicine. In today's class— *Basic Theory of TCM*, he learned five elements. He was puzzled by the fact that the five-element theory could be applied in diagnosis and treatment of disease, so he turns to his teacher doctor Wang and asks the teacher some questions.

Story Retelling

Cue Words

(1) 原理　theory, principle

(2) 地方官　local official

(3) 恶心　feel sick of sth.

(4) 弓　bow

(5) 影子　shadow

(6) 豁然开朗　be suddenly relieved

(7) 郁积的　pent

(8) 疑神疑鬼　be filled with suspicion

(9) 惊恐　fright

(10) 恐在五行中属水　fright is associated with water in five elements

(11) 心病还须心药医　whoever started the trouble should end it

杯弓蛇影

　　生活中的一些行为中往往也蕴含着中医五行生克的原理。有个成语叫"杯弓蛇影"，这个成语出自《晋书·乐广传》。晋代河南有个叫乐广的地方官，他有一个亲密的朋友，分别很久后不见再来，于是乐广就亲自上门去问朋友不来的原因。朋友回答说："前些日子到你家做客时，你请我喝酒，正端起酒杯要喝的时候，看见杯中有一条小蛇，心里十分恶心，但还是强忍着把酒喝下，喝了那杯酒以后，就得了重病。"乐广回家后思索这件事，他看到当时朋友坐着喝酒的座位旁边墙壁上挂着一张弓，弓上有一条漆画的蛇。乐广猜想朋友酒杯中的蛇一定是弓的影子，他再次请那位朋友来家里，并让他还在原来坐的地方饮酒，对朋友说道："酒杯中是否看见什么？"朋友回答说："所看到的跟上次一样。"于是乐广告诉了朋友酒杯出现蛇的原因。朋友听完后心情豁然开朗，疑团顿时解开，长久郁积的重病顿时治好了。这个故事后来变成了成语，比喻那些疑神疑鬼、自相惊扰的人。这个故事里还包含着一个用五行生克治病的道理。朋友喝了有蛇的酒被吓出了病，是为惊恐，恐在五行中属水，乐广解开朋友的心结靠的是思考，思在五行中属土，五行中土克水，情志上思克恐，因此"杯弓蛇影"的故事中包含着五行相克的道理，说明心病还须心药医。

Group Task

On the basis of the characteristics of five elements, the ancient thinkers made analogies between certain properties and functional characteristics of various things and phenomena. For example:

- Wood: flourishes and promotes growth.
- Fire: hot with warming and ascending actions.
- Earth: having generating, transmitting, carrying and receiving actions.
- Metal: having clearing, descending and astringent actions.
- Water: being cool, cold, moist, and moves downwards.

The five-element theory is mainly used to analyze the physiological functions of the viscera, meridians and their interconnections via the engendering and restraining relationships of the five elements. And it can be used to explain the viscera's physiological functions and their relationships. In TCM, the five *zang*-organs corresponds to the five elements, therefore we use the properties of the five elements to explain the physiological functions of these organs. For example, wood corresponds to the liver, and the nature of wood is growing freely, so the liver likes to be unrestrained and up-bearing but dislikes to be depressed.

Oral Task

Use five-element theory to talk about seasons, colors, orientations and flavors. Each group should choose one of the topics above and present your oral report in PPT.

Reading and Question Answering

Huoshenshan and *Leishenshan* Hospitals in Wuhan

The names of Wuhan's two new hospitals for combating the deadly new virus, *Huoshenshan* and *Leishenshan*, demonstrate Chinese people's connections to the country's traditional God of Fire and God of Thunder.

Huoshenshan Hospital, a 1,000-bed hospital with a quarantine area of 34,000 square meters, was put into use on Monday, while construction of *Leishenshan* Hospital, which has 1,300 beds, will be completed on Wednesday. *Huoshenshan* means Mountain of the Fire God, while *Leishenshan* means Mountain of the Thunder God.

God of Thunder

Worship of thunder gods is an ancient and global cultural phenomenon. It is the most widely worshiped type of god, according to a report of the Paper.

In China, the Thunder God is the god of punishment. Those who violate human ethics and commit unforgivable crimes will be struck to death by a bolt of lightning.

The images of the god changed throughout the centuries according to Chinese historical records and ancient murals. According to Mountains and Seas, a book recording ancient myths that was completed before the Qin Dynasty (221BC-206BC), the earliest image of the Thunder God has human head but a dragon's body.

After the Han Dynasty (206BC-AD220), the image of the god turned into a strong man who was half-naked.

Like Thor, the god of thunder in Norse mythology, the Chinese Thunder God also held a weapon in hands, but the difference is Thor possesses the magic hammer Mjolnir while the Chinese god uses a circle of drums and an awl to produce thunder and lightning.

In a mural of a royal noble's tomb from the Northern Dynasties, the God of Thunder is encircled by 13 drums. He looks as if he is stepping on different drums in the wall painting, and the drums continued to whirl under the furious taps, giving off a continuous and startling roar, according to the Paper.

The image of the Thunder God has always been muscled, strong-willed and furious in Chinese fairy tales, so the name was chosen for the hospital because it is believed it can suppress and defeat the deadly virus.

God of Fire

Huoshenshan Hospital's name is not only related to the ancient Chinese god but also contains elements of the Chinese philosophy of *Wuxing*, also known as Five Elements, which covers the five types of energies that become dominant at different times.

The five elements are metal, wood, water, fire and earth. In traditional Chinese medicine, each of these are also linked to the body's five major organs and are used to describe the interaction between these organs.

These five elements have two relations: mutual generation and mutual overcoming. Depending on the pairing, a certain element can help or give birth to another element and can also suppress a different one.

"In Traditional Chinese Medicine, metal represents the lungs. In *Wuxing*, fire overcomes metal," a Chinese medicine doctor Duan in North China's Shanxi province told the *Global Times* on Tuesday.

"I think the hospital's name contains fire to suppress the lung infection caused by novel coronavirus."

"The novel coronavirus is also vulnerable to high temperatures, so I think this is a good name," Duan added.

The Chinese God of Fire, also known as Zhurong, is described as the invincible nemesis of the God of Plagues in Chinese mythology as he can drive diseases away.

Zhurong is also said to be an ancestor of the eight lineages of the royal families of the Chu State of the Warring States (475BC-221BC). The state of Chu was located in the area that is today's Central China's Hubei province, where the virus originated.

Questions

(1) Search for information about the God of water and earth and make a short report.

(2) Can you give more examples of the use of five elements in daily life?

V Creative Oral Activity

Activity 1

There once was a newly elected mayor who came to a village to help the people. Being a newcomer, he met many challenges in governing the village and was overwhelmed by his heavy workload. Soon, he experienced severe pensiveness and felt very sick. One day, he turned to a renowned village doctor for help. The doctor firstly took his pulse and then thought for a while. Suddenly, he had a crazy idea and said, "Congratulations, mayor! Your symptoms are signs of pregnancy. Don't worry too much. You will get better soon." No sooner had the doctor spoken, the mayor shouted angrily, "Get out! I am male. How can I be pregnant? How ridiculous you are!" A short time later, the mayor's illness disappeared, just as the doctor had predicted. Can you use the theory of five elements to explain this?

Activity 2

The Use of Five Elements in Daily Life

Have you ever noticed the examples of using five-element theory in our daily life?

You are asked to collect the examples of the application of five-element theory in people's daily life. The following example is for your reference.

Example 1

In the comedy movie *Detective Chinatown 2*, James Springfield— a serial killer is fascinated by the five-element theory in TCM, and he mistakenly believes that if he kills five people based on five-element theory and Chinese astrology, using five kinds of *zang*-organs of those victims to practice alchemy, he could become immortal, and bring his dead wife back to life. However, the smart detective figures out the habit of the serial killer and successfully stops the killer from killing the last victim.

Example 2

In TCM, the universe is made up of five elements that reflect into the body via five organic systems. Chinese people believe that food therapy is a reliable and effective method to attain physical balance and cure illnesses and diseases.

TCM categorizes food based on colors and flavors so as to help people cook healthy and balanced meals based on the five-element theory.

Chapter Five

Qi, Blood and Body Fluids

Learning Objectives

In this chapter you will learn:
- The importance of *qi*, blood, and fluids for human health;
- Relative expressions on the given topic;
- A series of conversational expressions on the given topics.

I Lead-in Questions

(1) What's your understanding of *qi* from the angle of an average person?

(2) How many kinds of *qi* can you name (you may not have to answer it from the perspective of TCM)?

(3) What are the functions of *qi* in our body?

(4) How do you understand the Chinese expression that "body fluids and blood share the same origin" ?

II Useful Expressions

New Words and Phrases

(1) sweat /swet/ *n.* the salty colourless liquid which comes through your skin when you are hot, sick, or afraid 汗

(2) saliva /sə'laɪvə/ *n.* the watery liquid that forms in your mouth and helps you to chew and digest food 唾液

(3) urine /'jʊərɪn/ *n.* the liquid that you get rid of from your body when you go to the toilet 尿

(4) secrete /sɪ'kriːt/ *vt.* to produce a liquid substance 分泌

(5) insomnia /ɪnˈsɒmniə/ *n.* the condition of being unable to sleep 失眠（症）

(6) mucous membrane /ˌmjuːkəs ˈmɛmbreɪn/ *n.* a mucous membrane is skin that produces mucus to prevent itself from becoming dry, it covers delicate parts of the body such as the inside of your nose 黏膜

(7) orifice /ˈɒrɪfɪs/ *n.* (formal) (humorous) a hole or opening, especially one in the body（尤指身体上的）孔；穴；腔

(8) lubricate /ˈluːbrɪkeɪt/ *vt.* to put a lubricant on sth. such as the parts of a machine, to help them move smoothly 给 …… 上润滑油

(9) bladder /ˈblædə(r)/ *n.* an organ that is shaped like a bag in which liquid waste collects before it is passed out of the body 膀胱

(10) anatomy /əˈnætəmi/ *n.* the scientific study of the structure of human or animal bodies 解剖

(11) humor /ˈhjuːmə(r)/ *n.* 体液

(12) humor desertion 脱液

(13) liquid /ˈlɪkwɪd/ *n.* a substance that flows freely and is not a solid or a gas, for example water or oil 液体

(14) denote /dɪˈnəʊt/ *vt.* to be a sign of sth. 标志；预示

(15) stasis /ˈsteɪsɪs/ *n.* (formal) a situation in which there is no change or development 停滞

(16) impairment /ɪmˈpeəmənt/ *n.* the state of having a physical or mental faulty（身体或智力方面的）缺陷，障碍，损伤

(17) replenish /rɪˈplenɪʃ/ *vt.* (with sth) to make sth. full again by replacing what has been used 补充；重新装满

(18) extravasate /ɪkˈstrævəˌseɪt/ *vi.* to cause (blood or lymph) to escape or (of blood or lymph) to escape into the surrounding tissues from their proper vessels 使（血液或淋巴液等）从脉管中渗出

(19) speckle /ˈspekl/ *n.* a small coloured mark or spot on a background of a different colour 斑点；色斑

(20) palpable /ˈpælpəbl/ *adj.* that is easily noticed by the mind or the senses. 易于察觉的

(21) soot /sʊt/ *n.* black powder that is produced when wood, coal, etc. is burnt. 油烟

(22) vexation /vekˈseɪʃn/ *n.* the state of feeling upset or annoyed. 烦恼；恼火

(23) prenatal *qi* 先天之气

(24) postnatal *qi* 后天之气

(25) original *qi* 元气

(26) food *qi* 谷气

(27) nutrient *qi* 营气

(28) defensive *qi* 卫气

Sentence Patterns

(1) Life is the proliferation of *qi*, death its dissolution.

(2) If *qi* condenses, its visibility becomes effective and physical form appears.

(3) The ancient Chinese described *qi* as "life force".

(4) The *qi* of human body originates from three resources: innate *qi* (from kidney essence), acquired *qi* (formed by nutrients from spleen and stomach), and clear *qi* (air from lung) .

(5) Movement of *qi* includes upward, downward, inward and outward directions.

(6) Nutrient *qi* and body fluids and humor form blood.

(7) Fluid and humor include fluids within viscera and bowels, tissues and normal secretions. They are two types of body fluids that originate from dietary intake and depend on transporting and transforming function of the spleen and stomach.

(8) According to Chinese medicine, the formation of *qi* is closely related to the functions of the kidney, spleen, stomach and lung.

(9) Fluid is clear and thin. It moves easily and locates at skin, muscle, pores, and vessels. Moistening is its function. Humor is turbid and thick. It hardly moves and locates at tissues. Nourishing is its function.

III Model Dialogues

Conversation 1

Teacher: Good morning, Lucy.

Lucy: Good morning, Mr. Liu.

Teacher: Firstly, let's review the previous lesson. So, what are fluids?

Lucy: Well, "fluid" is a basic term in the theory of Chinese and it refers to all the normal fluid substances in the human body except for blood, such as sweat, saliva, stomach juices, urine, and other fluids secreted by or discharged from human body.

Teacher: Great! Can you talk about the features and functions of fluids?

Lucy: Well, fluids are clear and thin and they flow like water. Examples of fluids are tear, sweat and urine. They are distributed in the skin, muscles and orifices. They nourish the tissues and organs of human body.

Teacher: The next question is: "where do the fluids come from?"

Lucy: Body fluids are actually the watery substances transformed from the food and drinks we consumed everyday. They are transported by kidneys and lungs to all parts of human body through meridians and vessels.

Teacher: Do you know the differences between "fluid" (*jin*) and "humor" (*ye*)?

Lucy: Well, like what I said, fluid is like water, so it is relatively thin, moveable, and yang in nature, while humor is thicker, less moveable and yin fluid. Another difference is that fluid and humor can be found in different locations. For example, fluid exists in the skin, muscle and orifices, while humor exists in viscera, marrow and joints.

Teacher: Good answer. I am satisfied with your performance.

Lucy: Thanks for your praise, sir.

Conversation 2

Doctor: What's the matter with you?

Patient: Doctor, I always feel thirsty and dry in my throat. My lips and skin are dry, and there is no luster on my skin. My urine is scary and yellow and my defecation is dry.

Doctor: Does this situation last for a long time?

Patient: Yes, I have been like this all year round for a couple of years. At first, I didn't pay attention to it, but gradually I notice that there must be something wrong with my health.

Doctor: Yes, you are right. Possibly, you are suffering from the deficiency of fluids. But I still need to do further checking. Let me have a look at your tongue.

Patient: My tongue is red and I don't have much saliva.

Doctor: Any other symptoms?

Patient: Well, I often have palpitation and nightmares.

Doctor: They are the common symptoms of heart yin deficiency. In traditional Chinese medicine, heart maintains the normal functions of the vessels and meridians, and it governs people's mental activities. Since heart needs the nourishment from yin fluids, the lack of them would affect the functioning of the heart, leading to symptoms like palpitation, night sweat, insomnia, dreaminess and so on.

Patient: What should I do to change my current situation?

Doctor: Don't worry. We should first try to find out the reasons before I prescribe the right medicine.

Patient: Yes, that's right.

Doctor: How do you think about your living habits? I mean do you have any bad living habits?

Patient: Well, I am a taxi driver, so I often burn the midnight oil. And I like eating hot and spicy food.

Doctor: You need to change those bad living habits. Try to keep early hours and eat some food that is cool by nature. I will make a list of suggested food for you later on. And I will prescribe some medicines that can nourish your yin fluids and supplement the functions of your heart.

Patient: That sounds good, doctor. Thank you very much.

IV Oral Practice

Situational Dialogues

Situation 1

Jack and Tom are students from the College of Chinese Medicine, and they come to China for study because they were both fascinated by Chinese *Kongfu* TV dramas when they were kids, especially *Qigong* (breathing exercise). They are talking about *qi* in Chinese culture.

Situation 2

Blood is the red fluid circulating through the blood vessels, nourishing and moistening the whole body. Since blood is so important for health, Lucy, an exchange student from USA, is going to buy some food to nourish her blood. And you are a student majoring in Chinese medicine and you give her some suggestions.

Story Retelling

Cue Words

(1) 蹊跷　feel strange about sth.

(2) 丧事　funeral

(3) 江湖骗子　swindler

(4) 浮屠　pagoda

(5) 鼻翼　nose wing

(6) 大腿内侧　inner thigh

(7) 侍从　attendant

(8) 石针　stone needle

(9) 胁腹　flank

(10) 调理身体　to nurse one's health

(11) 尸厥　dead syncope

(12) 救人一命，胜造七级浮屠　To rescue one person from death is better than to build a seven-storied pagoda for the god.

起死回生

有一次，神医扁鹊路过虢国，见到全国上下都在祈祷，打听后才知道是虢国的太子在今天清晨鸡鸣时突然死了。

扁鹊打听了太子的症状，觉得太子死得蹊跷，为了一探究竟，便向一位负责太子丧事的官员请示，想去检查一下太子的死因，看看是否还有生还的希望。

太子的侍从认为扁鹊是江湖骗子，就冷嘲热讽一番说："你在开玩笑吧，人死了还能救活？连小孩都不会相信的。"救人一命胜造七级浮屠，扁鹊见侍从不信任自己，很是着急，多耽误一刻便会白白葬送一条人命。于是他灵机一动，对侍从说："你要是不相信我的话，那么你可以去看看太子，他的鼻翼一定还在扇动，他的大腿内侧一定还是温暖的。"

侍从半信半疑地将此话告诉了虢国大王，大王派人检查虢太子的尸体，发现果真如扁鹊所说。于是忙把扁鹊迎进宫中，痛哭流涕地说："久闻你医术高明，今日有幸得你相助。不然，我儿子的命就算完了。"

扁鹊一面安慰大王，一面命弟子磨制石针，针刺太子头顶的百会穴。不一会儿，太子竟渐渐苏醒过来，扁鹊又让弟子子豹用药物灸其两胁，太子便能慢慢地坐起来。后经过中药的进一步调理，二十来天后虢太子就康复如初了。

原来，虢太子并没有真的死亡，而是患了一种叫"尸厥"的病。扁鹊治好了尸厥，虢太子也就苏醒了过来。能让死去的人复活，真是让人大开眼界，这件事也很快被传遍各地，扁鹊走到哪里，哪里就有人说："他就是那个令人起死回生的神医啊！"以后，人们常用"起死回生"这个词来形容大夫的高超医术，也用来比喻把已经没有希望的事物挽救回来。

Group Task

Qi, blood, body fluids and essence are the basic substances in the human body, and they are also the material basis for the physiological functions of organs, tissues, meridians etc.

The elements of *qi*, blood and body fluids are closely related with each other and have the relationship of generating and being generated.

(1) Relationship between qi (yang) and blood (yin)

a. *Qi* can generate blood.

b. *Qi* controls blood circulation.

c. *Qi* promotes blood circulation.

d. Blood carries *qi* and supplies nutrients to it.

(2) Relationship between *qi* and fluid and humor

a. *Qi* generates fluid and humor.

b. *Qi* transports and transforms fluids and humor.

c. *Qi* controls fluid and humor.

d. Fluid and humor carry *qi*.

(3) Relationship between blood, fluid and humor

They all belong to yin, and are derived from food and have moistening or nourishing functions; meanwhile, they can transform to one another.

Oral Task

Work with your partners, and conduct an investigation to find out the reasons why nowadays many people lack *qi* and blood. Then, put forward suggestions about how to replenish *qi* and blood. Each group needs to assign a representative to give a 3-minute report.

Reading and Question Answering

Qi, Blood and Body Fluid

Qi, blood and body fluid are the basic substances that constitute the human body and maintain life activities. Their production and metabolism depend on the functional activities of the viscera, channels, organs and tissues.

i. *Qi*

Qi in TCM is the most essential substance to constitute the human body and sustain its life activity. *Qi* in the body is derived from innate qi that is transformed from the kidney essence inheriting from parents, and acquired *qi* from both food nutrients that are transformed by the spleen and stomach and fresh air that is inhaled by the lung. The production of *qi* depends on the synthetic actions of the viscera, especially the kidney, spleen, stomach and lung. *Qi* is powerful in activity and flows constantly in the body to maintain the physiological functions of the body. Such a constant motion of *qi* is called *qi* movement. The styles of *qi* movement are theoretically summarized as ascending, descending, exiting and entering. The viscera and meridians are the places where the activities of *qi* take place. According to the composition, distribution and functions, *qi* is mainly divided into four categories, namely primordial *qi*, pectoral *qi*, nutrient *qi* and defensive *qi*.

There are mainly five physiological functions of *qi*. The first is promoting. *Qi* is a vigorous and refined substance with powerful activity. It promotes and stimulates the growth and development of the human body, physiological activities of the viscera and meridians, the production and circulation of blood as well as the production, distribution and excretion of body fluid. The second is warming. *Qi* is the source of energy of the body.

This is prerequisite to the maintenance of normal body temperature, normal physiological activities of the viscera and normal circulation of blood and body fluid. The third is defending. The defending system of the body is in the body surface will consolidate the striae and interstices to prevent invasion of exogenous pathogenic factors. Under abnormal conditions, healthy *qi* can fight against pathogenic *qi*, driving it away to cure disease. The fourth is consolidating. *Qi* can prevent blood from extravasation and regulate the secretion and excretion of sweat, urine, saliva, gastric juice, intestinal juice and sperm in order to avoid unnecessary loss. The fifth is transforming. This action refers to the metabolism and mutual transformation of essence, *qi*, blood and body fluid. For instance, the production of *qi*, blood and body fluid depends on the transformation of food into nutrients; body fluid is converted into sweat and urine by means of metabolism; after digestion and absorption, the residues of food are turned into feces. All these processes are the concrete manifestations of the transforming action of *qi*.

ii. Blood

Blood is a red liquid substance rich in nutrients and circulating in the vessels. It is one of the indispensable materials to form the human body and maintain its life activities. Blood is mainly composed of nutrient *qi* and body fluid which come mainly from food nutrients transformed by spleen and stomach. That is why the spleen and stomach are considered as the source of *qi* and blood and play an important role in the production of blood. Since the nutrient *qi* and body fluid come from the nutrients of the foodstuff, the quality of food and the functions of the spleen and stomach directly influence the production of blood. Besides, the essence stored in the kidney is also an essential substance to promote blood production. That is why it is said that "the essence and blood share the same origin."

The main physiological function of the blood is to nourish and moisten the whole body. The blood circulates inside the vessels throughout the body, internally to the viscera and externally to the skin, muscles, tendons and bones. It flows continuously and ceaselessly to nourish and moisten all the organs and tissues to maintain their normal physiological functions. The nourishing and moistening functions of the blood are signified by such manifestations as ruddy complexion, well-developed and strong muscles, lustrous skin and hair, nimble and flexible sensation and movement. Blood is also the material basis for the mental activities. Therefore it is said in *Ling Shu* that "the harmony of blood and smoothness of the vessels are key to the normal state of the spirit."

iii. Body fluid

Body fluid is a collective term for all kinds of normal liquids in the body, including secreta from various organs and tissues, such as gastric juice, intestinal juice, nasal discharge, tears, sweat and urine, etc. Body fluid is derived from the foodstuff mainly transported and transformed by the spleen and stomach. According to the difference in property, function and distribution, it is subdivided into two *jin* (thin fluid) and *ye* (thick fluid). Generally speaking, thin fluid mainly spreads in the skin, muscles and orifices, and penetrates into the vessels as a component part of blood while thick fluid mainly maintains in the skeleton, joint, viscera and brain. Nevertheless, fluid and the liquid are of no difference in nature, so they are often collectively termed as "body fluid".

The production, distribution and excretion of body fluid is a complicated physiological process involving multiple viscera. The physiological functions of body fluid include moistening and nourishing the body, transforming and enriching blood, regulating yin and yang, neutralizing toxin and excreting waste. *(Excerpted from TCM English(《中医英语》2nd Edition) by Li Zhaoguo and Zhang Qingrong. The book was published by Shanghai Science & Technologies Publishers in September, 2013. This article is on page 78~80.)*

Questions

(1) What are the differences among primordial *qi*, pectoral *qi*, nutrient *qi* and defensive *qi*?

(2) What are the functions of blood in TCM?

(3) What are the differences between *jin* and *ye*?

V Creative Oral Activity

Qi, blood, and body fluids are fundamental substances of the human body which sustain the normal physiological functions of the *zang-fu* organs and tissues. However, in this fast-paced society, many people are under huge stress and they always complain that they are deficient in *qi* or blood.

Introduce 1-2 prescriptions that can supplement *qi* and blood, illustrate the usage and dosage.

Are there any good herbs that can supplement *qi* or blood in your local area? If yes, please introduce them to your classmates.

Chapter Six

Visceral Manifestation

Learning Objectives

In this chapter you will learn:

● The technical terms related to the theory of visceral manifestation;

● Situations where visceral manifestation are talked about;

● A series of conversational expressions related to visceral manifestation.

I Lead-in Questions

(1) Can you point out the places of five *zang*-organs in a human body?

(2) Do you know the differences between five *zang*-organs and six *fu*-organs?

(3) What are the different understandings of the concept of heart between Western medicine and Chinese medicine?

II Useful Expressions

New Words and Phrases

(1) viscera /ˈvɪsərə/ *n.* the large organs inside the body, such as the heart, lungs and stomach 内脏

(2) manifestation /ˌmænɪfeˈsteɪʃn/ *n.* an event, action or thing that is a sign that sth. exists or is happening; the act of appearing as a sign that sth. exits or is happening 显示, 表明

(3) bowel /ˈbaʊəl/ *n.* the tube along which food passes after it has been through the stomach, especially the end where waste is collected before it is passed out of the body 肠

(4) extraordinary organs 奇恒之腑

(5) triple energizer /ˈenədʒaɪzə(r)/ 三焦

(6) five body constituents /kənˈstɪtʃʊənts/ 五体

(7) pericardium /ˌpɛrɪˈkɑːdɪəm/ *n.* the membranous sac enclosing the heart 心包

(8) gallbladder /ˈɡɔːlˌblædə(r)/ *n.* 胆囊

(9) small intestine /smɔːl ɪnˈtestɪn/ *n.* 小肠

(10) bladder /ˈblædə(r)/ *n.* 膀胱

(11) uterus /ˈjuːtərəs/ *n.* [解剖] 子宫

(12) orifice /ˈɒrɪfɪs/ *n.* 孔口

(13) visceral manifestations 藏象

(14) blood chamber 血室

(15) five *zang*-organs and six *fu*-organs 五脏六腑

(16) transmitting and transforming water and food 传化水谷

(17) storing essence 贮藏精气

(18) internal and external relationship 表里关系

(19) therapeutic effects 治疗效应

(20) clinical practice 临床实践

(21) store without excrete 藏而不泻

(22) excrete without storage 泻而不藏

(23) physical build and various orifices 形体诸窍

(24) open at 开窍于

(25) spirit and emotions 精神情志

(26) the heart storing spirit 心藏神

(27) the lung storing corporeal soul 肺藏魄

(28) the liver storing ethereal soul 肝藏魂

(29) the spleen storing reflection 脾藏意

(30) the kidney storing will 肾藏志

(31) five *zang*-organs: heart, liver, spleen, lung and kidney 五脏

(32) six *fu*-organs: the small intestine, large intestine, gallbladder, bladder, stomach and triple energizer 六腑

(33) extraordinary organs: brain, marrow, bone, vessel, gallbladder and uterus 奇恒之腑

(34) five body constituents: sinews, vessels, flesh, skin and bones 五体

Sentence Patterns

(1) The theory of visceral manifestation studies the physiological functions and pathological changes of viscera and their relations.

(2) The common physiological functions of the five *zang*-organs are to transform and store essence.

(3) The common physiological functions of the six *fu*-organs are to receive, transport and transform water and food.

(4) Disorders of the five *zang*-organs are often of deficiency type in nature while disorders of six *fu*-organs are of excess type in nature.

(5) Excess of five *zang*-organs can be treated by purging the corresponding bowels while deficiency of six *fu*-organs can be treated by reinforcing the related viscera.

(6) The physiological functions of the five *zang*-organs play a leading role in the physiological functions of the whole body.

(7) Disorder of spirit, emotions and mental activity affects the physiological functions of the five *zang*-organs.

(8) The theory of visceral manifestation is based on the knowledge of anatomy in ancient times.

(9) The physiological functions of the heart are to govern blood and to control the mind.

(10) The heart can propel blood to circulate within the vessels, which relies on the propelling and warming functions of heart *qi* and heart *yang* as well as the nourishing and moistening functions of heart-yin and heart-blood.

(11) In a broad sense, spirit refers to the supreme dominator of life activities in the whole body. In a narrow sense, spirit is a collective term for cognition, thinking, consciousness and mental state.

(12) The heart opens into the tongue, so the state of the tongue can reflect the physiological functions and pathological changes of the heart.

(13) The heart has its external manifestation on the face.

(14) The heart and the small intestine are internally and externally related to each other.

(15) The lungs are located at the highest position among all the internal organs, so they are compared to a "canopy".

(16) The physiological functions of the lungs are dominating *qi* and managing the regulation of water passage.

(17) Water passage refers to the route for transmitting and discharging water. The lungs governing the regulation of water passage refers to the function of the lungs in propelling, adjusting and discharging water.

(18) The lungs govern the skin, which on the one side means the lungs can disperse and transport the *Wei Qi* (defensive *qi*) and body fluid to the skin to warm, nourish and moisten the skin so as to maintain the normal functions of the skin; on the other side, it means the lungs control the normal opening and closing activities of the sweat pores.

(19) The lungs open into the nose which is an sensory organ for air to be breathed in

and out of the body.

(20) The lungs have their external manifestation on the body hair.

(21) The liver has two functions: to govern *Shu Xie* (dredging and regulating) and to store blood.

(22) The liver governs *Shu Xie* actually means that the liver dredges the routes and regulates the movement of *qi* so as to ensure the smooth flow of *qi* in the body.

(23) The liver governs the tendons which are the tissues that connect the muscles, the skeleton and the joints.

(24) The liver opens into the eyes, so the eyesight is closely related with the liver. Insufficiency of liver-yin and liver-blood may lead to dryness of the eyes and blurred vision, failure of the liver to dredge and regulate may lead to up-flaming of liver fire, bringing on redness, swelling and pain of the eyes and cataract.

(25) The liver has its external manifestation on the nails. The nails are believed to be extensions of the tendons and they depend on liver-blood to nourish, so the insufficiency of liver-blood often affects the color and quality of the nails.

(26) The spleen, located in the abdomen, governs transportation and transformation and to command blood.

(27) When food is taken into the stomach, it is digested and absorbed by the stomach and the small intestine, but it must depend on the transporting and transforming functions of the spleen to transform the food into nutrients which are distributed to the four limbs and other parts of the body.

(28) The spleen controls blood circulation inside the vessels and prevents it from flowing out of the vessels.

(29) The spleen governs the muscles and the four limbs. It means the muscles and the four limbs depend on the nutrients transported and transformed by the spleen to nourish.

(30) The spleen has its external manifestation on the lips.

(31) The physiological functions of the kidney are to govern growth and development, to govern reproduction, to govern water, to govern reception of *qi*, to produce marrow and to nourish and warm the internal organs.

(32) The kidney stores essence, *qi*, yin and yang. The human growth mainly depends on the kidney-essence, kidney-yin and kidney-yang.

(33) The kidney governs the bones, which means that the development and functions of the bones depend on the kidney-essence.

(34) The kidney opens into the ears, the external genitals and the anus.

(35) The kidney has its external manifestations on the hair.

III Model Dialogues

Conversation 1

Jack: I was told that Chinese medicine can tell the visceral conditions by observing a person's external appearance.

Li Ming: Yes, you're right. Based on the Theory of Zangxiang (visceral manifestation), the physiological and pathological changes of the internal organs can be reflected via external signs on human body, orifices and sensory organs.

Jack: I understand. It embodies the philosophical concept of association. For example, heart is associated with the tongue and it has its external manifestation on the face.

Li Ming: Wow. I can't believe you know so much about visceral manifestation.

Jack: In fact, I just know some basic information about it. I am by no means a scholar on Chinese medicine, but I have to say I am truly interested in it. Oh, by the way, can you help to check my body? I feel that something is wrong with my heart.

Li Ming: Why do you think so?

Jack: Well, look at my tongue. It is always pale and whitish. And look at my face, blackish with no luster. I guess my heart-qi and blood is insufficient.

Li Ming: Yes, I agree with your judgment. Just as the saying goes, "The tongue is the sprout of the heart" , and heart opens at the tongue, which makes the tongue a mirror to reflect the condition of the heart.

Jack: Then, what should I do to cope with this problem?

Li Ming: First, you need to lead a healthy lifestyle. I mean that you should keep regular hours and try to avoid mood swings.

Jack: Yes, staying up late truly damages my health. I will go to sleep early from today on. What else?

Li Ming: Take herbal medicines which can supplement *qi*, such as ginseng, *Huangqi* (Radix Astragali), red jujube, and Chinese yam.

Jack: Thank you for your suggestions.

Conversation 2

Lily: I am so worried about my health after learning the lesson on visceral manifestation.

Jack: What's the matter with you?

Lily: I guess there is something wrong with my stomach.

Jack: Why do you say so?

Lily: Well, based on the theory of visceral manifestation in Chinese medicine, stomach has the function of receiving and digesting food, and it is called the "Sea of Food and Drinks". The stomach-*qi* should move downward smoothly. If it moves upward, there will be symptoms like nausea, vomiting and belching with gastric acid. According to the *Huangdi's Internal Classic*, "When the patient's stomach is in disorder, he can not lie down and sleep well." It seems that I have all the symptoms.

Jack: Come on, don't be so serious. You can not say that you have problems with your stomach simply because you once in a while displayed those symptoms.

Lily: But I truly often have stomachache and constipation? And I have bad breath.

Jack: There is no doubt that your external manifested symptoms are related with stomach problems. In this case, you really need to have a check on your stomach.

Lily: Yes, the lesson on visceral manifestation is truly useful. Although it does not provide cure or prescriptions for my health problems, it can help me detect those problems before they get worse.

Jack: Yes, you are right. And you do it simply by observation, which saves you the fees of medical examination, but to do further and in-depth examination, you still need to seek professional help from doctors.

IV Oral Practice

Situational Dialogues

Situation 1

Madam Wang is coughing badly recently, so she went to see a doctor yesterday. She went to a local clinic of Chinese medicine. After inquiry and diagnosis, the doctor said that her illness was caused by her low mood and sadness. The fact is that Madam Wang is very tired of taking care of her son, and her husband is working in the United States, so she actually could only rely on herself, thus she is unhappy all the time. However, she cannot figure out the relationship between her cough and her mood. Now you will play the role of the doctor and explain the whole thing for her.

Situation 2

The five *zang*-organs, namely heart, liver, spleen, lung and kidney, argue fiercely with each other over who is the most important organ to their master. Please prepare a comedy, and six students are needed to play the roles of the five *zang*-organs and the master himself.

Situation 3

Jack comes from the USA and he is now studying in Jiangxi University of Chinese Medicine as an exchange student. He is very interested in learning Chinese medicine; however, he has a lot of puzzlement. For example, he finds it difficult to understand the different connotations of five *zang*-organs in TCM. You are Jack's classmate and you help him understand the meanings and functions of five *zang*-organs in Chinese medicine.

Story Retelling

Cue Words

(1) 相传　legend has it that
(2) 装神弄鬼　be deliberately mystifying
(3) 巫医　witch doctor
(4) 膏肓　Gaohuang (inter cardiodiaphragmatic part)
(5) 膈　diaphragm
(6) 病入膏肓　a disease that is beyond cure

病入膏肓

相传，晋国的君主晋景公生病，他先请来装神弄鬼的巫医为自己治疗，病情反而有增无减。于是，他派人到秦国求医。秦国派了一位名叫医缓的医生去给他治病，医缓的高明医术全国上下无人不知。

当医缓还在去晋国的路上时，晋景公梦见从他的病中跳出两个小人，其中一个说："医缓是医术高明的医生，可不比前次那个巫医，他恐怕要抓住我们，该往哪里躲避呢？"另一个回答说："到心的下面、膈的上面，叫'膏肓'的那个地方去吧，看他能把我们怎么样？"医缓到了晋国，给晋景公辨证后为难地说："这病不可治啦！病在膏肓，不能采取攻伐的治法，何况药物也不能到达那里去发挥药效。"

后来，人们常用"病入膏肓"形容病情严重，难以医救。这句话进一步引申时便用来形容一个人犯错误到了不可挽救的地步。

Group Task

The content of *Zang Xiang* theory is composed of three parts: the physiological functions and pathological changes of the viscera, the description of which mainly focuses on the physiological functions; the relationships between the five *zang*-organs and the body, organs and orifices, including the relationships between the five *zang*-organs and the five constituents (namely vessels, tendons, muscles, skin and bones), the five sensory organs and the nine orifices (namely the tongue, eyes, mouth, nose, ears, external genitals and anus); the relationships between the *zang*-organs and the *fu*-organs, including the relationships among the five *zang*-organs, among the six *fu*-organs and the relationships between the *zang*-organs and the *fu*-organs.

You are asked to work with your partners and search for the relationship between five *zang*-organs and five constituents and the orifices, as well as the external manifestations of five *zang*-organs on special areas (ie. the face, the body hair, the tendons, the lips and the hair).

Reading and Question Answering

The Five *Zang*-organs

The five *zang*-organs include the heart, lung, spleen, liver and kidney, among which the heart is the dominant one. Therefore, it is said in *Su Wen* that "the heart is the monarch organ".

The heart is situated in the thorax, above the diaphragm and enveloped by the pericardium. Its meridian connects with the small intestine with which it is internally and externally related. The main physiological functions of the heart are to control the blood and vessels and govern the mind. It opens into the tongue, manifesting on the face, associating with joy in emotions and sweat in secretion.

Spirit is an important conception in TCM. In a broad sense, spirit refers to the outward manifestations of the life activities; in a narrow sense, it refers to mental activities, including spirit, consciousness and thinking, etc. The theory of *zangfu* organs holds that thinking is related to the physiological functions of the heart. For that reason, spirit, consciousness, thinking and memory are all related to the function of the heart in storing the spirit. Therefore, *Ling Shu* says that "the heart is the residence of the spirit". Blood, which is controlled, dominated and regulated by the heart, is the main material basis for the mental activities. So, normal physiological function of the heart to control the spirit will ensure full vitality and consciousness, agile mind and normally sensitive reactions to the external stimulation. However, the abnormal changes of the physiological function of the heart in storing spirit will bring on such symptoms as insomnia, dreaminess, distraction and even delirium, or slow reaction, amnesia, dispiritedness and even coma.

The heart opens into the tongue. When the functions of the heart are normal, the tongue will be rosy, moist and lustrous in color, normal and sensitive in taste, free and flexible in movement. The disorders of the heart, on the other hand, will also be reflected on the tongue. For example, if yang *qi* in the heart is insufficient, the tongue will appear light-colored, whitish, bulgy and tender; if the blood is deficient in the heart, the tongue will appear deep-red, thin and dry; if the heart fire flames up, the tongue will appear reddish or even with ulcer; if the heart vessels are stagnant, the tongue will appear cyanotic or even with ecchymoses; if the physiological function of the heart in controlling the spirit is abnormal, the tongue will become curled and stiff.

The lung, including two lobes on the left and right, is situated in the thorax, communicates with the throat and opens into the nose. The lung is compared to the "canopy" because of the uppermost position among all the viscera. Its meridian is internally and externally related to the large intestine. The main physiological functions of the lung are to dominate *qi* and control respiration, govern ascent, dispersion, purification and descent as well as regulate water passage. The lung is related to sorrow in emotions and the skin and hair in the exterior. The lung opens into the nose.

The spleen is located in the middle energizer and below the diaphragm. Its meridian connects with the stomach with which it is externally and internally related. The main physiological functions of the spleen are to govern transportation and transformation, control blood and dominate muscles and limbs, open into the mouth and associate with thought in emotions and slobber in secretion.

The liver is located in the right hypochondriac region below the diaphragm in the upper abdomen. The liver meridian connects with the gallbladder with which it is internally and externally related. The main physiological functions of the liver are to store blood, govern free flow of *qi*, control tendons and open into the eyes.

The liver not only stores the blood, but also regulates the volume of blood in circulation. For this reason, the liver is closely related to all the activities of the viscera and tissues. So deficiency of liver blood may lead to such symptoms as blurred vision, spasm and convulsion of the tendon sand muscles, numbness of the four limbs, and oligomenorrhoea or even amenorrhoea in women. The liver is closely related to emotional activities. That is why dysfunction of the liver is frequently accompanied by emotional changes such as mental depression or excitement.

The kidney is situated at either side of the lumbus. The main functions of the kidney are to store essence, control growth, development and reproduction, govern water, receive *qi* and open into the ears, anus and urethra. The kidney also dominates the bone and manufactures marrow. The kidney meridian connects with the bladder, with which it is internally and externally related.

Questions

(1) What are the physiological functions of the heart?

(2) What is the relationship between heart and spirit?

(3) What are the physiological functions of the lungs?

(4) What are the physiological functions of the spleen?

(5) What are the symptoms of a person who suffer from liver blood deficiency?

V Creative Oral Activity

Portable Aromatic Oxygen Generator

Lily is now a student from Jiangxi University of Chinese Medicine. She is majoring in Chinese medicine. Last week she attended a lecture introducing aroma therapy which is a special treatment using herbs with fragrant smells to treat diseases. Commonly used herbs are clove, agasthche, costustoot, angelica root, mint, borneol and musk.

Aroma therapy is an ancient medical therapy dating back to thousands of years ago. At first, it was invented by Egyptians who extracted essential oil by soaking fragrant plants and then used the oil in the process of massage in order to nourish their skin.

In China, aroma therapy has its earliest records in pre-Qin period when it was used as a medical treatment to deal with certain diseases. In the Zhou Dynasty, people had the habit of wearing perfume satchel and having hot bath in orchid-brewed water. In the book *Compendium of Materia Medica* compiled by Li Shizhen, detailed description about aroma therapy can be found.

In modern society, aroma therapy has improved a lot. And there are various ways of administrating the herbs, such as essential oils, smoking and spray. Based on TCM theory, aroma therapy has the function of regulating *qi* movement in viscera and bowels and restoring the yin and yang balance in human body, thus helping patients maintain health.

In clinic treatment, aroma therapy is used to treat sleeping problems, mood disorders, postoperative vomiting (POV), gynecological diseases, skin diseases and so on.

Lily was highly impressed by the lecture and a creative idea occurred to her. And she was going to invent a device which combines the oxygen production and aroma therapy. She called it portable aroma oxygen generator(移动香氧).

She plans to inject essential oils extracted from medical herbs into humidified container(湿化瓶), and then oxygen will bring the essential oils into lungs. This device can treat different kinds of diseases by putting different essential oils into the container, and it can also serve the purpose of disease prevention.

Oral Task

Lily is going to tell her ideas to her teacher Mr. Zhang and her teacher likes the idea. Please make up a dialogue between Lily and Mr. Zhang.

Chapter Seven

The Four Diagnostic Methods

Learning Objectives

In this chapter you will learn:
- Professional terms associated with the four diagnostic methods of TCM;
- Conversational skills on four diagnostic methods.

I Lead-in Questions

(1) What are the four kinds of diagnostic methods in TCM?

(2) What are the approaches for doctors to determine a patient's condition?

(3) What's the possible problem with a person who has grayish and dark face?

II Useful Expressions

New Words and Phrases

(1) auscultation /ˌɔːskəlˈteɪʃn/ *n.* the process of listening to sb's breathing using a stethoscope 听诊

(2) olfaction /ɒlˈfækʃən/ *n.* the sense of smell 嗅觉

(3) palpitation /ˌpælpɪˈteɪʃən/ *n.* [内科] 心悸

(4) acupuncturist /ˈækjʊpʌŋktʃərɪst/ *n.* an acupuncturist is a person who performs acupuncture 针灸师

(5) fluid /ˈfluːɪd/ *n.* a liquid; a substance that can flow 液体，流体

(6) puffy /ˈpʌfɪ/ *adj.* if a part of someone's body, especially their face, is puffy, it has a round, swollen appearance 圆肿的

(7) metabolize /məˈtæbəlaɪz/ *vi.* to turn food, minerals, etc. in the body into new cells, energy and waste products by means of chemical processes 新陈代谢

(8) deficiency /dɪˈfɪʃnsi/ *n.* the state of not having, or not having enough of, sth (sth.) that is essential 缺乏；不足

(9) excess /ɪkˈses/ *n.* more than what is necessary, reasonable or acceptable 过度

(10) stagnation /stæɡˈneɪʃn/ *n.* 停滞

(11) subtle /ˈsʌtl/ *adj.* not very noticeable or obvious 不易察觉的，微妙的

(12) patterns identification 辨证

(13) dissipate /ˈdɪsɪpeɪt/ *vi.* to gradually become or make sth. become weaker until it disappears（使）消散；驱散

(14) influenza /ˌɪnfluˈenzə/ *n.* influenza is the same as flu 流行性感冒

(15) inspection, observation, looking 望诊

(16) listening and smelling, auscultation and olfaction 闻诊

(17) inquiry, questioning, history taking 问诊

(18) pulse taking and palpation, feeling the pulse 切诊

(19) synthesis of the four diagnostic methods 四诊合参

(20) have bright eyes 眼睛有神

(21) bad breath 口臭，口中异味

(22) distinguished features of TCM 中医特色

(23) *cun*, *guan* and *chi* 寸、关、尺

(24) examine the tongue 看舌

(25) spleen-heart deficiency 心脾两虚

(26) pathological conditions 病理状态

(27) tongue coating 舌苔

(28) spirit / vitality / mental activity 神

(29) complexion 面色

(30) physical build 体形

(31) postures and physical movements 态

(32) life activities 生命活动

(33) loss of spirit 失神

(34) sufficiency of essence and *qi* 精气足

Sentence Patterns

(1) The four diagnostic methods-inspection, listening and smelling, inquiry and pulse taking and palpitation-are the basis of syndrome differentiation and treatment.

(2) Observing a patient's appearance could help TCM doctors discover the pattern and development of his illness.

(3) Loss of spirit causes death while maintenance of spirit ensures life.

(4) The human body is an organic whole. Local pathological changes may affect the

viscera and the whole body and can be detected from the manifestations of the sensory organs, limbs and surface of the body.

(5) Inspection of the exterior manifestations will enable one to understand the interior conditions; diagnosis of the exterior manifestations will enable one to know the interior states.

III Model Dialogues

Conversation 1

Jack: I find that the four diagnostic methods applied in Chinese medicine really aroused my interest.

Li Ming: Where did you get to know it?

Jack: I experienced it myself. I mean, I saw a doctor of Chinese medicine yesterday because of my stomach problem, and the way he diagnosed me was so different from the practice of Western medicine. I know you major in Chinese medicine, so can you tell me more about this oriental diagnostic method?

Li Ming: Well, that will be a long story to tell. But I can tell you that the four diagnostic methods have a long history and they are widely used by doctors of Chinese medicine. They are believed to be invented by Bian Que in the Warring States period.

Jack: I know Bianque, the legendary miracle-working doctor in Chinese medicine. And what are exactly the four diagnostic methods?

Li Ming: They refer to inspection, auscultation and olfaction, inquiry and pulse-taking.

Jack: Well, I guess the doctor who diagnosed me yesterday used the four methods, because he observed my face and tongue, smelled my breath and took my pulse.

Li Ming: Yes, a doctor of Chinese medicine can gather the first-hand information about a patient's disease with the four diagnostic methods.

Jack: But what puzzles me is how can the doctor know the situation of my stomach by observing my face or tongue?

Li Ming: Well, that is the method of inspection. A doctor can get hold of the information about a patient's disease by inspecting the patient's facial color, mental state, physical posture, tongue, skin and excrement, etc.

Jack: What problems with my stomach do you see by looking at my face and tongue?

Li Ming: Well, I am not so professional as the doctor you saw yesterday, but I guess you may have digestive problem based on my inspection.

Jack: Amazing! Your judgement is exactly the same as the doctor diagnosed. He said that I got dyspepsia, which means that the digestive function of my stomach is poor. How do you make your diagnosis?

Li Ming: Well, quite simple. Your face is sallow yellow, and your lips are whitish, which show that you're having malnutrition and this is often caused by the dysfunction of the stomach. And your tongue coating is thick and white, which often originates from dysfunction of the spleen and the stomach, thus confirming my judgment.

Jack: Wow. You really surprise me. Thank you for your explanation.

Conversation 2

Li Ming: Hi, Jack. I didn't see you in yesterday's TCM class. How dare you skip professor Wang's class?

Jack: I didn't. I mean I've asked for his permission. I had a important matter to attend to yesterday. Anyway, what do I miss yesterday? I'll have to make it up.

Li Ming: The part of auscultation and olfaction of the four diagnostic methods.

Jack: Oh, I see. It refers the practice of diagnosing diseases by listening to the sounds and smelling odors giving off by the patient, right?

Li Ming: Yes, it seems that you have grasped what I learnt yesterday. No need to make up anything.

Jack: No, I know only a thing or two about it. Can you tell me more?

Li Ming: Well, we listen to the sound made by the patient to know whether he is suffering from a deficient or excess syndrome. For example, if a patient speaks with sonorous and forceful voice, he possibly suffers from yang or heat syndromes.

Jack: That's unbelievable. How can it be possible to diagnose a patient simply by listening to his voice?

Li Ming: Of course, it can't. The method of auscultation is a part of a complicated diagnosis system. I mean, it is aided with other methods like inspection, inquiry and pulse-taking.

Jack: Yes. That really makes sense. A patient with yang or heat syndromes would have symptoms like reddish face, feverish body, vexation, feeling of thirst, yellowish tongue coating, etc.

Li Ming: This method even applies to patients who do not make any sounds?

Jack: I don't see what you mean.

Li Ming: Well, there are two situations right here. The first one is that the patient makes hoarse voice, and the other is that the patient cannot utter any sound no matter how hard he tries.

Jack: I know the reason why a patient makes hoarse voice lies in the yin deficiency and exuberant fire, which in turn cause the lack of yin fluid in the lungs and kidneys and the throat loses its nourishment. As to aphonia, the situation where a patient cannot make sound, it is either due to the excessive use of throat or the exhaustion of qi in five-*zang* viscera after lengthening illness.

Li Ming: Your analysis really impresses me. But, I have to go now. Next time I'd like to go on with this topic about the part of smelling.

Jack: Thanks, Li. Catch you later!

IV Oral Practice

Situational Dialogue

Situation 1

Lily is an exchange student from the USA. She is very interested in the tongue diagnosis in TCM, but she has a lot of puzzlement, so she turns to Wang Ming—her classmates for help. Wang Ming will introduce the theory and practice of tongue diagnosis in TCM to Lily. The following picture (pic. 1) illustrates the correspondence between five *zang*-organs and the tongue.

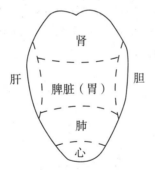

Pic. 1 Correspondence of five *zang*-organs on the tongue

Reference for tongue diagnosis

- Teeth marks on the tongue: spleen deficiency and heavy dampness.
- Pale white tongue: lack of *qi* and blood.
- Tongue coating mottled: inadequate spleen and stomach *qi*.
- Lack of tongue coating at the base of the tongue: deficiency of kidney *qi*.
- The tongue is thickly coated: retention of food in stomach.
- Tongue coating covers the tongue body:excessive dampness, phlegm and retained fluid.

- Red spots on the tongue: heat in the body.
- Black spots or dark purple spots on the tongue: blood stagnation.

Situation 2

A patient is now visiting doctor Wang. The patient has the following possible chief complaints:

- light fever
- severe aversion to cold
- spells of fever and cold at the same time
- runny nose and frequent sneezing
- headache and body pain

Try to make a dialogue between the patient and the doctor based on the above situation by using the four diagnostic methods.

Situation 3

Jack comes from the UK and he is very interested in traditional Chinese medicine, because he has experienced the magical treatment of TCM when he was in London. Today, he is visiting the campus of Jiangxi University of Chinese Medicine. He heard that there were many interesting stories about the four diagnostic methods in ancient China, such as Bian Que visiting Cai Huan Gong. You are asked to be the guide during his stay in your university, and since he is so interested in stories about four diagnostic methods, you are asked to tell him one of those stories.

Story Retelling

Cue Words

(1) 医圣 medical sage
(2) 祠堂 memorial temple
(3) 疑神疑鬼 be extremely suspicious
(4) 巫婆 witch
(5) 鬼怪缠身 be haunted by ghosts
(6) 驱邪 to drive out evil spirits
(7) 气色 complexion
(8) 热入血室 heat entering blood chamber
(9) 扎针 apply acupuncture

张仲景看气色驱"魔"

张仲景从小爱好医学，年轻时曾跟同郡的张伯祖学医。经过多年的刻苦钻研和临床实践，张仲景医名大振，成为中国医学史的杰出医学家。他一生为民医病，深受老百姓爱戴。后来人们尊称他为医圣，在南阳城东关修了一座"医圣祠"来纪念他。

有一次，张仲景遇见一个妇女，她一会儿哭一会儿笑，总是疑神疑鬼。病人家属听信巫婆的欺骗，以为这是"鬼怪缠身"，要请巫婆为她"驱邪"。张仲景观察了病人的气色和病态，又询问了病人的有关情况，然后对病人家属说："她根本不是什么鬼怪缠身，而是'热血入室'，是受了较大刺激造成的。她的病完全可以治好，真正的鬼怪是那些可恶的巫婆，她们是'活鬼'，千万不能让她们缠住病人，否则病人会有性命危险。"在征得病人家属同意后，他研究了治疗方法，为病人扎了几针。几天后，妇女的病慢慢地好起来，疑鬼疑神的症状也消失了。张仲景又为她治疗了一段时间，她就痊愈了。

Group Task

The four diagnostic methods are widely used in Chinese medicine to help doctors to get a comprehensive understanding about a patient's pathogenic and physiological conditions. You are asked to illustrate the use of four diagnostic methods in medical practice with concrete examples.

Reading and Question Answering

The Diagnosis Database

When 66-year-old Xi Lipin recently went to a community hospital in Pudong New Area for a traditional Chinese medicine (TCM) treatment, the exam went off without a hitch.

Like always, she opened her mouth so her tongue could be examined and held out her wrist so her pulse could be taken. Twenty minutes later, she received a printout with her symptoms and suggested treatment.

The examination was similar to every other TCM examination Xi has ever gotten, except this time it was done by a computer.

The computer, called the Household Digital TCM-Four Diagnostic Apparatus, can handle most basic forms of TCM examination. Since last month, it has been used to help doctors diagnose patients at Shanggang Community Health Service Center in Pudong.

The machine demonstrates the efforts that researchers are putting into making TCM more scientific and more in line with mainstream medical care around the world. The hope is that the machine will help promote TCM, which lacks credibility outside of East Asia and is considered alternative medicine in the west due to the dearth of evidence about its efficacy.

"With the computer, we try to standardize and digitalize the TCM diagnosis process," said Wang Yiqing, a professor at the Shanghai University of Traditional Chinese Medicine, who helped develop the machine. "It is the first step toward getting it accepted by more people, so we can promote it."

Digital diagnosis

This computer, which was also on display at the 2010 World EXPO in Shanghai, has three main parts: a digital camera to scan patients' faces and tongues, a device for checking pulses, and a screen that asks patients 70 questions, primarily about their symptoms. After collecting the information, the computer will analyze the patients' answers and compare them to a database in order to make a diagnosis.

The system is designed to diagnose patients with the four main diagnostic methods of TCM-Wang, Wen, Wen and Qie (inspection, auscultation and olfaction, inquiry and pulse-taking).

TCM treats the body holistically. Practitioners believe that internal problems can be discerned in the complexion, voice, pulse and tongue texture. By analyzing these indicators, doctors can learn what is wrong with their patients.

"At first, it was just a curiosity," said the patient Xi. "But after experiencing it, I think the system is scientific. It acts like a normal TCM doctor, and the descriptions of the symptoms are quite accurate."

The accuracy of the systems depends on the database, which is a collection of years of TCM diagnoses. "We've collected more than 40,000 diagnoses, with each verified by at least two TCM experts," Wang said.

The machine is not designed to replace a doctor. "It's like an X-ray machine in Western medicine. It provides doctors with important information. But it cannot work alone."

Building the machine

This computer is the result of years of work by TCM researchers to apply technology to their discipline. "The biggest advantage of these pieces of equipment is to objectify and standardize TCM," said 62-year-old Su Minliang, who has been a TCM doctor for 40 years. "Traditionally, the TCM diagnosis is based on doctors' subjective observations. So, for the same patient, different doctors may have different conclusions. And those conclusions may also be influenced by a doctor's mental and physical state. Because of that problem, TCM treatments sometimes seem unreliable."

Su said the new technology can offset this problem to some extent. "For example, an experienced doctor can take a patient's temperature by touching his forehead, but he can't be as accurate as a thermometer. "

Since 1997, Su has been using an electronic pulse-taking device that he helped design in his hospital in Beijing. For TCM practitioners, feeling a patient's pulse can tell them far more than the patient's heart rate.

He said the machine has won the trust of many patients. "Its accuracy has been shown after years of use. Every day, around 70 patients go to see this digital doctor, " he said. "With its help, young doctors can make diagnoses without a lot of experience. "

TCM computers are also expected to play an important role in recording and passing down the experience of senior TCM doctors.

"In the past, the TCM theories were like old folk songs. They are recorded and taught in a language that fewer and fewer people can understand. Therefore, to standardize it is essential for its future development, " Wang said.

'A long way to go'

Still, after 14 years, Su's pulse-checking machine is still used in only one hospital. "It proved successful in a town in Shanxi province in 2008. However the local government rejected it since it led to the unemployment of several TCM doctors there," Su said. "I think it will take time before the market is prepared for such machines."

Su also worries the technology will prevent young TCM doctors from completely learning the craft. "It takes years to learn TCM's methods for diagnoses, such as feeling the pulse. But with a machine, one doctor can acquire that ability without any effort. However, if one day no doctors master the most basic TCM practice, how can it be improved?"

Some patients are also critical about introducing technology into TCM, fearing TCM will eventually lose something with digitalization.

"I personally cannot accept computerized TCM, " said a 56-year-old patient surnamed Cheng, who has been seeing TCM doctors for more than five years. "You can't call it TCM after it has been computerized. If I choose to trust some figures and indexes, why not choose Western medicine? After all, they have far more advanced machines."

Some doctors point out that the machines are quite limited. "TCM is holistic so it is not about A leading to B. For the same diseases, we may use different treatments for different patients. So I doubt current computers are clever enough to adopt that diagnostic process," said Zhou Duan, a TCM doctor with more than four decades of experience.

Wang admitted that there is a lot of room for computerized TCM to improve. "We plan to add a new function to diagnose patients through their odor and voice-one of the four diagnostic methods 'Wen' - so as to make it more trustworthy," she said. "But it's just one step forward in modernizing TCM. We have a long way to go."

Questions

(1) Do you think the four diagnostic practice will be replaced by machine someday in the future?

(2) What is your expectation for the improvement of machine on diagnosis?

V Creative Oral Activity

Lily, an American western doctor, has always been interested in TCM. Recently she watched a Chinese TV drama called *Journey to The West*, in which one scene aroused her strong interest in the four diagnostic methods of TCM. That is when the Monkey King pretended to be a doctor and attached three strings to the wrist of the king's daughter in order to examine the patient's condition. Lily was surprised by the magical oriental medical skills and she wants to know more about it, so she turns to doctor Wang who is a doctor of Chinese medicine.

Please make up a dialogue based on the given situation.

Chapter Eight

Treatment Based On Syndrome Differentiation

Learning Objectives

In this chapter you will learn:
- Professional terms related with this treatment principle in TCM;
- A series of conversational expressions and skills on a given topic.

I Lead-in Questions

(1) What are the differences between the ways of diagnosing diseases in Chinese and Western medicine?

(2) How do you understand the Chinese proverb "*Tou Tong Yi Tou, Jiao Tong Yi Jiao*" (to treat only where the pain is)?

II Useful Expressions

New Words and Phrases

(1) syndrome /ˈsɪndrəʊm/ *n.* a set of physical conditions that show you have a particular disease or medical problem 综合征

(2) differentiation /ˌdɪfəˌrenʃiˈeɪʃn/ *n.* 辨别

(3) bloated /ˈbləʊtɪd/ *adj.* full of liquid or gas and therefore bigger than normal, in a way that is unpleasant 膨胀的

(4) nauseous /ˈnɔːziəs/ *adj.* feeling as if you want to vomit 恶心的

(5) regurgitation /rɪˌɡɜːdʒɪˈteɪʃn/ *n.* 回流

(6) appetite /ˈæpɪtaɪt/ *n.* physical desire for food. 食欲；胃口

(7) bowel /ˈbaʊəl/ *n.* the tube along which food passes after it has been through the stomach, especially the end where waste is collected before it is passed out of the body 肠

(8) barium /ˈbeəriəm/ *n.* 钡

(9) prolapse /ˈprəʊlæps/ *n.* a condition in which an organ of the body has slipped forward or down from its normal position（身体器官的）脱垂

(10) diabetes /ˌdaɪəˈbiːtiːz/ *n.* a medical condition caused by a lack of insulin , which makes the patient produce a lot of urine and feel very thirsty 糖尿病

(11) bout/baʊt / *n.* an attack or period of illness（疾病的）发作

(12) interior syndrome 里证

(13) eight principles (exterior and interior, cold and heat, deficiency and excess, yin and yang）八纲（中医）

Sentence Patterns

(1) Exterior pattern is characterized by sudden onset, aversion to cold or wind, fever, headache, general pain, thin tongue coating, and floating pulse.

(2) Patients who suffer from exterior pattern may have symptoms like nasal congestion, runny nose, sneezing, sore throat and cough.

(3) Internal damage can be caused by seven emotions, overexertion, fatigue, improper diet, sexual overindulgence, and injury.

(4) Interior patterns are usually manifested by the symptoms and signs of diseases of the viscera and bowels, *qi* and blood, fluid and humor.

(5) Half-exterior half-interior pattern is due to affliction located between the exterior and interior of the body, marked by alternate fever and chills, fullness and choking feeling in the chest, bitter taste in the mouth, dry throat, nausea and loss of appetite, and string-like pulse.

(6) Cold pattern is a general term for patterns caused either by external cold pathogen or by insufficient yang within the body, commonly manifested by aversion to cold or fear of cold, cold pain with preference for warmth, absence of thirst, thin clear sputum and nasal mucus, long voiding of clear urine, loose bowels, whitish complexion, pale tongue with white coating, and tight or slow pulse.

(7) Heat pattern is a general term for patterns resulting either from attack of external heat or from prevalence of *yang qi*, usually manifested by fever, aversion to heat and liking for cold, thirst, flushed face, irritability and vexation, thick yellow sputum and nasal mucus, short voiding of dark-colored urine, constipation, reddened tongue with yellow coating, and rapid pulse.

(8) Deficiency pattern is usually manifested by fatigue, lack of strength, shortness of breath, no desire to speak, spontaneous sweating, loose stool, emaciation, pain alleviated by pressure, vexing heat in the chest, palms and soles, tidal fever, flushed cheeks, night sweating, pale or swallow complexion, palpitation, withered skin, tender tongue with

scanty fur and weak pulse.

(9) Excess pattern is a general term for patterns caused by external pathogenic factors such as six climatic factors, pestilential pathogens, worms and toxins. Excess pattern can also be caused by accumulated pathological products due to dysfunction of internal organs, such as phlegm, retained fluids, water, dampness, pus, static blood and retained food, and usually manifested by high fever, delirium, chest oppression, heavy breathing, profuse sputum and drool, abdominal pain and/or tenderness and refusal of pressure, tenesmus of dysentery, stranguria, tough tongue with thick or slimy fur and replete pulse.

III Model Dialogues

Conversation 1

Li Ming: Are you having cold, Jack? Your voice is hoarse and I can see that you have nasal obstruction.

Jack: Yes, I guess so. But don't worry about me. It's a minor illness, and I will just buy some medicines for cold in the pharmacy.

Li Ming: Well, you'd better see a doctor of Chinese medicine and get the right medication.

Jack: I don't think it's that serious.

Li Ming: Well, the case is you haven't done syndrome differentiation and you may possibly take the improper medicine, which in turn worsens your situation.

Jack: I don't see what you mean. Are you talking about things on Chinese medicine?

Li Ming: Yes, based on traditional Chinese medicine, cold or flu can be classified into either the excess or deficient type.

Jack: What is excess type cold?

Li Ming: Well, the excess type cold refers to common cold due to wind-cold and wind-heat, and common cold caused by summer-heat and dampness. They each have different symptoms and should be treated with different medicines.

Jack: What about cold of deficient type?

Li Ming: This refers to the cold caused either by *qi* or *yin* deficiency. *Qi* deficiency often leads to lengthened and repeated cold, and this often happens on old people and children who are physically weak. Menopausal women often suffer from cold of yin-deficient type.

Jack: Wow, I have never thought that a common cold can be divided into so many different types. Then which type of cold suits my situation?

Li Ming: That can be diagnosed from your symptoms?

Jack: Well, I have splitting headache, chest distension and I feel uncomfortable in my stomach. I have no desire for food and feel so weak all over the body.

Li Ming: What about your tongue? Show me. The coating is slightly reddish. So I can say that you are probably suffering cold caused by summer heat and dampness. Did you eat anything iced or raw?

Jack: Yes, I ate iced watermelon yesterday.

Li Ming: Well, that's the thing to blame.

Conversation 2

Doctor: Good morning, what's the matter with you?

Patient: Doctor. I have a terrible headache. It has tortured me for quite a long time.

Doctor: Don't worry. Let me have a look at your tongue and take your pulse.

Patient: I don't mean to offend, doctor. What's the use of looking at my tongue and feeling my pulse since my problem is in my head?

Doctor: Well, I understand your confusion. Let me explain it for you. Headache is caused either by pathogens invading the exterior or by internal damage. The former refers to situations when wind, heat or dampness invades us through the exterior, while the latter refers to headache caused by exuberant liver fire or kidney deficiency.

Patient: Sorry, doctor. Please excuse me for being impolite. I have never though that the reasons for headache are so complex.

Doctor: That's all right. I can only give you the right prescription after I figure out the cause for your situation, right?

Patient: Yes, that's right.

Doctor: Well, you have reddish complexion, thin and yellowish tongue coating, and your pulse is rapid and robust. Do you feel bitterness in your mouth?

Patient: Yes, I often feel bitterness in my mouth.

Doctor: Do you sleep well at night?

Patient: No. I often have insomnia or bad dreams, I mean, I become violent and upsetting in the dreams.

Doctor: Are you easy to get agitated?

Patient: Well, yes. I confess I am a guy of bad temper. I may become very angry over trivial things, and sometimes I am so angry that my belly would be painful.

Doctor: Based on diagnosis, your headache is caused by excessive liver fire. And I will prescribe some medicines to nourish your liver. However, it is equally important for you to keep peaceful, for mood swing would worsen your situation.

Patient: Thank you, doctor. I will do it.

IV Oral Practice

Situational Dialogues

Situation 1

Lily is suffering from sleeping problems recently. She is talking to Xiaohui who is a student majoring in TCM. The following information is for your reference.

(1) There are a couple of reasons for insomnia, such as mental stress, spendging time on the phones till deep night, diseases and noisy environment.

(2) As explained by Chinese medicine, insomnia can be caused either by diseases, such as coughing, anxiety, abdominal pain, etc., or by disharmony of yin and yang, *qi* and blood.

(3) Due to the increasing pressure of modern life, many people may get stagnation of liver *qi*, which would in turn becomes liver fire flowing upward to brain, thus causing sleeping trouble.

(4) Too much contemplation will lead to dysfunction of spleen and stomach, thus affecting the transporting and transforming of *qi* and blood, and human body and brain could not be nourished, which leads to insomnia.

(5) There are many effective TCM therapies for insomnia. For example, massage *Yongquan, Taixi* and *Shimian* those three acupoints for 3-5 minutes a day; take formulas such as *Anshen Buxin Wan* (Nerve-calming Heart-invigorating Pill); eat food that is good for sleeping, such as red date, longan, apple, banana, mulberry kernel and milk.

Situation 2

Hans is in the school canteen and he is having dinner with his Chinese friend Li Ming. Li Ming notices that Hans has no appetite, so he asks about the situation. It turns out that Hans is having stomach problem. So Li Ming diagnoses him and gives him some medical suggestions. The following is for your reference.

(1) Hans has abdominal pain which can be alleviated by pressing and his tongue is whitish with greasy coating.

(2) His pulse is sunken and slow.

(3) Hans prefers warm drinking recently, and he feels like vomiting occasionally.

(4) Hans is diagnosed with stomach cold. The treatment is to warm the middle energizer and reinforce the function of stomach.

(5) Li Ming suggests stewing a pig stomach with ginger, which can dispel cold in

stomach and nourish the stomach.

Situation 3

Mrs. Li gets a cold. She feels very bad with nasal stuffiness, nasal discharge, sneezing and cough. She goes to see a TCM doctor. According to her symptoms, make up a dialogue with your partner, and play the roles as doctor and patient separately.

Story Retelling

Cue Words

(1) 成语　idiom
(2) 对症下药　suit the remedy to the case
(3) 诊断　diagnosis
(4) 药方　prescription/ recipe
(5) 发散药　herbs with dispersing function
(6) 泻药　herbs with purging function
(7) 伤食　indigestion

对症下药

东汉末年，有一位杰出的医学家叫华佗，他的医术非常高明。有两个病人，一个叫李延，一个叫倪寻，都得了头痛发热病，找过很多医生也没治好，于是来找华佗。华佗经过细心诊断，给他们各开了一个药方，给李延开的药方是发散药，给倪寻开的药方是泻药。他俩一看，心里就嘀咕起来：都是一样的病，怎么用药完全不同呀？便问华佗这是什么道理。华佗说："吃药要看具体情况，你们症状相同，可是得病的原因却不同。倪寻的病是从内部伤食引起的，李延却是从外部受寒造成的。病因不同，当然用药就不能相同了。"两人听了，便放心服药，病果然很快好了。这个故事就是成语"对症下药"的来源。

Group Task

Syndrome differentiation is one of the basic principles to diagnose and treat diseases. It was first proposed by Zhang Zhongjing, a physician in the Eastern Han Dynasty in his masterpiece called *Shang Han Za Bing Lun* (*Treatise on Cold-Attack and Miscellaneous Diseases*).

Differentiation means "discrimination". In other words, doctors should treat every patient differently by taking patients' physiological and pathogenic conditions into consideration, even though the patients are getting the same kind of disease.

Syndrome is the generalization of the progress of a disease at a certain stage, including various factors, such as the location and nature of the disease, the relation between pathogenic factors and healthy *qi*.

In clinical practice, syndrome differentiation can comprehensively and accurately reveal the nature of a patient's disease, which helps the doctor to give the corresponding therapy. Taken as a whole, syndrome differentiation is the process to understand and resolve a disease.

Discuss with your partner, and write a report on the enlightenment that syndrome differentiation gives to you.

Reading and Question Answering

Northeast China's Jilin province reported 30 newly confirmed locally transmitted COVID-19 cases and 17 new asymptomatic cases on Jan 17, according to the Health Commission of Jilin province. The province has taken five measures to cope with the possible further increase in the number of confirmed cases.

There are 66 designated hospitals and 27 designated backup hospitals in Jilin province, with 6,881 beds available for COVID-19 treatment, including 709 intensive care beds. At present, all confirmed cases and asymptomatic cases are receiving isolated medical treatment at these designated hospitals.

The provincial expert group is divided into six regional sub-groups. Each sub-group is responsible for the consultation and treatment of confirmed cases in two regions to ensure that every COVID-19 patient in the province has access to provincial-level expert consultation and treatment guidance.

Jilin is making full use of the experience of its medical teams that supported Wuhan last year to provide high-quality healthcare services for patients. It is planning to set up a provincial medical squad and increase the practical training of medical institutions at all levels.

Jilin also fully utilizes its five top hospitals and carries out the centralized allocation of medical resources. The five leading hospitals at the provincial level are responsible for treatment of critically ill patients in specific areas.

The province adheres to integrating traditional Chinese medicine (TCM) and Western medicine, the principle of "one person, one prescription" and the standardized use of drugs. All confirmed cases and asymptomatic cases are being treated according to syndrome differentiation.

At the same time, the concept of disease prevention is followed, and preventive use of TCM is carried out for all close contacts and sub-close contacts of COVID-19 patients at centralized quarantine stations.

Questions

1. What are the advantages of giving patients treatment based on syndrome differentiation?

2. Are there any possible drawbacks on syndrome differentiation?

V Creative Oral Activity

Many stories about syndrome differentiation show the miracles of Chinese medicine. For example, Xiong Jibai, a renowned National TCM Master from central China's Hunan province, once shared his experience about syndrome differentiation as follows: "I remember, 3 years ago, I treated a man who could not walk due to a car accident. Since his legs were slightly swollen, so the doctors who treated him all believed it was due to trauma of the accident. But the CT film of his legs showed that his bone fracture had cured. I observed the patient's legs and noticed that though his legs were mildly swollen, but no bruises were shown. Although it was difficult for him to walk, there was no difficulty for him to bend and straighten his legs. After making an inquiry, I know that he felt intermittent heat on his feet, bitter taste in the mouth and his urine was yellowish. And his tongue coating was greasy and yellowish and his pulse was soggy. Based on the diagnosis, I think he suffers from rheumatism caused by heat dampness and I thus prescribed *Er Miao San* Powder for him and he recovered ten days later."

Oral Task

You are required to prepare another story about syndrome differentiation like the above one.

Chapter Nine

Etiology
....

Learning Objectives

In this chapter you will learn:

● How to express the causes of diseases from the perspective of TCM;

● How to conduct conversations about cause of diseases from the perspective of TCM.

I Lead-in Questions

(1) Why do people get sick?

(2) What are the effects of climate changes on human bodies?

(3) Do you think emotions will lead to diseases? How?

II Useful Expressions

New words and Phrases

(1) etiology /ˌiːtɪˈɒlədʒɪ/ *n.* the etiology of a disease or a problem is the study of its causes 病原学

(2) taut /tɔːt/ *adj.* stretched tightly 绷紧的

(3) phlegm /flem/ *n.* the thick substance that forms in the nose and throat, especially when you have a cold 痰

(4) asthma /ˈæsmə/ *n.* asthma is a lung condition that causes difficulty in breathing 哮喘

(5) antibiotic /ˌæntɪbaɪˈɒtɪk/ *n.* antibiotics are medical drugs used to kill bacteria and treat infections 抗生素

(6) bronchitis /brɒŋˈkaɪtɪs/ *n.* bronchitis is an illness like a very bad cough, in which

your bronchial tubes become sore and infected 支气管炎

(7) diffuse /dɪˈfjuːz/ *vt.* if something such as knowledge or information is diffused, it is made known over a wide area or to a lot of people 传播（知识、消息等）；散布

(8) arthritis /ɑːˈθraɪtɪs/ *n.* arthritis is a medical condition in which the joints in someone's body are swollen and painful 关节炎

(9) exogenous /ɛkˈsɒdʒɪnəs/ *adj.* having an external origin 外源的

(10) internal damage 内伤

(11) damage to fluid 伤津

(12) overexertion /ˌəʊvərɪgˈzəːʃən/ *n.* 过劳

(13) overexertion and fatigue 劳倦

(14) pestilence /ˈpɛstɪləns/ *n.* pestilence is any disease that spreads quickly and kills large numbers of people 瘟疫

(15) pestilential *qi* 疠气

(16) flavor predilection /ˌpriːdɪˈlekʃn/ 五味偏嗜

(17) dietary irregularities 饮食失调

(18) traumatic injuries /trɔːˈmætɪk/ 外伤

(19) insect and animal bites 昆虫和动物咬伤

(20) six climatic factors（it refers to six kinds of external causes of diseases, namely, wind, cold, summer heat, dampness, dryness, and fire)

(21) seven emotions（it is a collective term for joy, anger, anxiety, thought, sorrow, fear and fright）

Sentence Patterns

(1) When summerheat attacks the human body, there will be high fever, sweating, flushed face, dry mouth, dizziness and vertigo.

(2) When attacked by dampness, the patient feels as if he were bearing a heavy load and he may have symptoms of a heavy head with the feeling of being swathed, heavy body, and sluggish or heavy limbs.

(3) Dryness injures the lungs and impairs body fluids. When human body is attacked by dryness, it is marked by thirst, scanty urine, dry cough, and scanty and sticky phlegm.

(4) Disease caused by fire is manifested by thirst with desire for cold drinks, tiredness, or mental disorder.

(5) Pestilential *qi* is a pathogen that causes epidemic infectious disease.

(6) According to the theory of five emotions in TCM, excessive anger causes damage to the liver, excessive joy or fright causes damage to the heart, excessive thought causes damage to the spleen, excessive sorrow or anxiety causes damage to the lungs, and excessive fear causes damage to the kidney.

(7) Anger causes *qi* to ascend. When anger is in excess, it may cause the liver *qi* to ascend together with blood, resulting in irritability, headache, dizziness, flushed face, bloodshot eyes, or hematemesis, even sudden fainting.

III Model Dialogues

Conversation 1

Li Ming: Hi Lily, you look worried. What's the matter with you?

Lily: Well, it's actually not me. It's my mom. She is so irritable recently.

Li Ming: Is your mom suffering from menopausal problems? That's normal for women of your mother's age.

Lily: I don't know what exactly the reasons are. She just suddenly became so bad-tempered to me after she had several nights without good sleep.

Li Ming: Do you know what leads to her sleeplessness?

Lily: She confessed that after knowing the happy news of my elder brother being admitted by Peking University, she was so overjoyed that she couldn't sleep any longer.

Li Ming: Well, I guess I have found out the reason for your mom's situation. Her mood swing was probably caused by what we called "internal damage due to emotional disorders".

Lily: What? You mean being overjoyed caused my mom's diseases.

Li Ming: Yes, you can understand it that way. Based on Chinese medicine, the reasons for diseases are various, such as six pathogenic factors, improper diet, pestilential *qi*, excess of seven emotions, and the like. So you will see that seven emotions, namely anger, joy, worry, thought, grief, fear and fright, are considered as one of the reasons for diseases.

Lily: But it is hard for me to correlate my mom's happiness with her changes in temper.

Li Ming: Let me explain it this way. Chinese medicine holds that people's emotions can have direct impact on five internal organs. For example, excessive anger damages the liver, and excessive joy damages the heart. There are too many examples showing that over joy may turn a normal person to be crazy.

Lily: But my mom didn't complain that she has anything wrong with her heart.

Li Ming: Well, in Chinese medicine, heart serves more functions than pumping blood all over the body. It also governs people's mind. So your mom's excessive joy damages her heart, and that's the reason why she couldn't fall asleep.

Lily: I start to see what you mean. Then, what can we do to help my mom?

Li Ming: First, you should do something to help your mom to maintain a calm mind, say, take her out for a short trip. Second, eating some food red in color could be helpful. For example, your mom are suggested to eat food like tomato, hawthorn, and jujube dates. Those foods can nourish the heart.

Lily: Thank you, Li Ming.

Conversation 2

Li Ming: Hi, Lily. What's the matter with you? It seems that your nose is stuffed up.

Lily: Yeah. Keep the distance with me. I may pass the infectious disease to you.

Li Ming: Why are so sure that your disease is infectious? Based on Chinese medicine, there are various types of cold, and the cold that is caused by virus is one of the five types of cold.

Lily: That sounds interesting! I thought cold was invariably caused by either virus or bacteria.

Li Ming: Well, Chinese medicine holds that there are mainly two reasons for cold: either the internal reasons or the external reasons. The former refers to the condition when a person's healthy *qi* is so weak that outward pathogenic factors invade. So when a person's healthy *qi* is strong enough, he won't get sick. Just as quoted in *Yellow Emperor's Canon of Medicine*, "When there is healthy *qi* inside the body, evils cannot invade".

Lily: You really impressed me. I have never thought you are so good at Chinese medicine. What about the external reasons?

Li Ming: External reasons refer to the six kinds of extreme climatic factors that invade human body, such as wind, cold, summer heat, dampness, dryness and fire, as well as seasonal pestilential *qi*.

Lily: No wonder you said that there were five types of cold. I guess the classification is based on the different reasons of cold, right?

Li Ming: And their different symptoms. For example, in spring when it is still chilly, people may get a cold that is called "wind-cold restricting the exterior". And patients who get this type of cold may have symptoms like headache, runny nose, nasal obstruction, and light fever. While in summer when it is hot, people may get a cold which is called "wind-heat type cold", and they may get different symptoms such as sore throat, sneezing, yellowish nasal discharge, thirst and vexation.

Lily: What is the type of my cold, then?

Li Ming: We have to find out the reasons before making decision. What symptoms do you have?

Lily: Well, I have this repeated cold with aversion to wind, fever, nasal obstruction, and I feel so weak that I don't even have the strength to breathe and I am unwilling to speak.

Li Ming: Come here and sit down. Let me feel your pulse. Well, it is quite weak.

Based on your own confession and symptoms, I can say your cold is caused by deficiency of *qi*. And you need to have some herbal medicine to supplement your middle *qi*. Formulas like *Shen Su Yin* (Decoction of Ginseng and Perilla Leaf) and *Bu Zhong Yi Qi Tang* (Decoction of Middle-*qi* Tonifying) are effective to relieve your situation.

Lily: Thank you, Li Ming.

IV Oral Practice

Situational Dialogues

Situation 1

Lily is recently suffering from a series of symptoms, such as carebaria (the feeling of heaviness in head), weakness of limbs, pain all over the body, joint stiffness, abdominal fullness and distension, nausea and vomiting, and loss of appetite. She confesses that she likes cold drinks, especially in hot summer days. Doctor Wang, a TCM practitioner, suggests her keeping doing exercise and adjusting her dietary habit after diagnosing her with body dampness and spleen deficiency.

Situation 2

A beautiful season though, spring is also a season when children are more possible to get flu and stomach diseases. Lily's son was down with heavy flu, so she took him to a TCM clinic where the doctor prescribed some herbs and gave her some disease-preventing suggestions after making a diagnosis that her son get the cold of wind-heat type.

Story Retelling

Cue Words

(1) 医术　medical skills
(2) 精于　be skillful in
(3) 诊断　diagnose
(4) 传播　spread
(5) 手到病除　bring health to patient immediately
(6) 小病　minor disease
(7) 针管放血，在皮肤上敷药　perform bloodletting by injecting tubes into vessels or applying medical ointment on the skin

扁鹊治未病

一天，扁鹊为魏文王治病之后，魏文王问扁鹊："你家中三个兄弟，都精于医术，自家三兄弟相比谁的医术更高？"

扁鹊答道："要是论医术，在我们三兄弟中，医术最好的就是我家大哥，次之就是我家二哥了，医术最差的就是我。"

魏文王接着问道："那为什么你最有名气呢？"

扁鹊答道："我家长兄给人家治病，是在病人发病之前就诊断出来了，经过他的治疗，病人很快就会康复。治病于病发之前，对于病人和病人家属来说，他们并不知道病人的病被提前诊断出来和治愈了，所以长兄的名气就无法向外传播。我二哥治病于人们患病初期，疾病在初期看上去还不那么严重的时候，就被我二哥手到病除了，人们以为我的二哥只会治疗微小的疾病呢，其实不然。我给患者看病的时候，一般都是病情比较严重的时候，患者和患者家人看到我在患者身上穿针管放血，在皮肤上敷药等，都以为我的医术高明，就把我的名声传遍全国了。"

Group Task

There are some commonly-seen diseases in people's daily life, such as influenza, fever, cough, acute gastroenteritis, oral ulcer, gastritis, etc. Work with your partners and search for possible reasons and solutions to three kinds of disease and make a short report.

Reading and Question Answering

The Yellow Emperor's Inner Canon-Just What the Doctor Ordered

Huangdi Neijing or *Huangdi's Internal Classic* is the earliest book on the theories and practices of traditional Chinese medicine. Compiled by several ancient Chinese doctors and medical scholars more than 2,300 years ago, it has been deemed one of China's top four medical classics and a cornerstone of Chinese medicine.

Most of the book's contents were written or compiled during the Warring States Period (475-221 BC), though one or two chapters are believed to have been put together during the early years of the Western Han Dynasty (206 BC-AD 25).

The work is composed of two parts, each containing 81 chapters. They are written in a question-and-answer format, recording conversations between the mythical Huangdi, or Yellow Emperor—the earliest ancestor of the Chinese nation, and his ministers, chiefly Qibo, a mythological Chinese doctor, and Shaoyu, a legendary acupuncturist.

The first part of the book is called *Suwen* or *Basic Questions* which discusses the nervous system, channels and collaterals, etiology, diagnostic methods, treatment principles and acupuncture.

The second part, called *Lingshu* or *Spiritual Pivot* focuses more on acupuncture therapy, acupoints, acupuncture methods and needling instruments, as well as acupuncture treatment principles.

In general, the book covers topics such as overall concepts of Chinese medicine, *yin* and *yang*, five elements— metal, wood, water, fire and earth—disease prevention and maintaining good health.

It describes a human being as a microcosm interacting with his or her surrounding natural conditions or the macrocosm. The key is to keep both the balance within one's microcosm and the balance between the microcosm and the macrocosm.

The book advocates preventive treatment and holistic therapy. It includes three steps: first, disease prevention; second, early diagnosis and prevention of disease progress; and third, prevention of disease recurrence and treating conditions that may follow an ailment.

It also lists many dos and don'ts in order to be healthy. For instance, the book advises people to be abstemious, eat more vegetables, keep a healthy lifestyle, seek peace of mind, be magnanimous and read books.

Huangdi's Internal Classic also asks readers to get enough sleep, because it could take more than 100 days to make up the loss of one night's sleep.

The book also warns of the bad effect of having sex after drinking alcohol and advises readers not to try to spit great a distance, saying this can sap vitality.

It also reminds readers to perform 10 drills: clicking the teeth; swallowing saliva; kneading the nose; stroking the ears; rolling the eyeballs; It is commonly known that there are different infectious diseases threatening human beings. For example, children are susceptible to disease like hand-foot-mouth disease, chickenpox, influenza and children pneumonia. And in different seasons, there are different epidemics, especially during the turn of seasons. For example, spring is the season when many epidemics may possibly break out, such as influenza, measles, chicken pox, mumps, rubella and scarlet fever. After having enough knowledge about the patterns of occurrence of different diseases, it is important for human beings to take actions beforehand. As we know, prevention is more important than curing. Take COVID-19 for example, in 2020 the occurrence of COVID-19 gave a heavy blow to the whole world, especially America where millions of people got this pandemic and tens of thousands of patients died of it. If Americans had taken actions in the early time of 2019, the situation would not be like this.

When it comes to disease prevention, TCM has long been known for its concept of *Zhi Wei Bing* (preventive treatment of disease), as is evidenced by the saying "The best measure is to treat the disease before it happens, not to cure disease" , a quotation from *Huangdi's Internal Classic*.

The theory of *Zhi Wei Bing* is mainly to advocate the idea and concept of prevention, and take corresponding measures to prevent the occurrence and development of diseases.

The following is a news report about the use of TCM preventive treatment in fighting against COVID-19. TCM is playing a part in fighting against COVID-19, even beyond China. In Mauritius, a country known as a gateway to the Indian Ocean where TCM doctors, while concerned with the epidemic's situation back in China, are figuring out a way for the control and prevention of the coronavirus in the locality.

Wang Xiaosu and Hu Binglin, two TCM doctors from Shanghai Yueyang Hospital of Integrated Traditional Chinese and Western Medicine, have been working at the China-Mauritius TCM Center since 2019, an institution founded last year in Port Louis, capital of Mauritius. After COVID-19 broke out in China, they have been in close contact with their colleagues who are now fighting at the frontline in Wuhan's *Leishenshan* Hospital. While learning from the Wuhan experience of fighting against the disease, they also wanted to help with preventing the virus spreading in Mauritius.

Mauritius is a tourist attraction for the Chinese during the Spring Festival, while many Chinese residents in Mauritius flew back to China to spend the holiday, so they need to be checked upon arriving back. Because of the poor prevention facilities in Port Louis and people's low awareness of the epidemic, if there is a single imported case of COVID-19 in the country, the consequences could be disastrous.

As such, Dr. Wang Xiaosu and Dr. Hu Binglin decided to prioritize the prevention of the epidemic in the China-Mauritius TCM Center. Upon learning that a tourist from Hubei was put under quarantine because of a fever and two staffers at the Chinese embassy felt discomfort at work, Wang and Hu prepared a lecture about the prevention, diagnosis and treatment of novel coronavirus pneumonia for the Chinese embassy and healthcare institutions in the locality.

Prevention and control play a crucial part in fighting infectious diseases. As COVID-19 has been deemed a global health emergency, the entire world has to stand in solidarity to fight the epidemic. Through the TCM center in Mauritius, Yueyang Hospital will work hand in hand with the Mauritian government and its people by sharing Chinese doctors' treatment experience through the integration of traditional Chinese medicine and western medicine.

V Creative Oral Activity

Oral Task

Task 1

You are required to prepare a presentation introducing the preventive methods against

COVID-19 by using TCM knowledge. Work with your teammates, and try to collect resources online.

Task 2

Prepare a report introducing the use of TCM treatments in fighting against COVID-19 in foreign countries.

Task 3

Prepare a presentation introducing the use of preventive treatment of diseases via TCM.

Chapter Ten

Acupuncture and Moxibustion

Learning Objectives

In this chapter you will learn:

● The professional terms on acupuncture;

● The conversational expressions and practice about acupuncture and moxibustion.

I Lead-in Questions

(1) Have you ever tried acupuncture or moxibustion? If yes, in what kind of situation did you undergo the treatment?

(2) What kind of ailments or disorders can be treated with acupuncture?

(3) Why does acupuncture treatment become more and more popular throughout the world?

II Useful Expressions

New Words and Phrases

(1) acupoints /ˈækjʊˌpɔɪnt/ *n.* 穴位

(2) gallop /ˈɡæləp/ *vt.* to ride a horse very fast, usually at a gallop（马）飞奔

(3) constitution /ˌkɒnstɪˈtjuːʃn/ *n.* the condition of a person's body and how healthy it is 体质，体格

(4) pediatric /ˌpiːdiˈætrɪk/ *adj.* 小儿科的

(5) efficacy /ˈefɪkəsi/ *n.* the ability of sth., especially a drug or a medical treatment, to produce the results that are wanted（尤指药物或治疗方法的）功效

(6) register /ˈredʒɪstə(r)/ *vt.* to record your/sb's/sth's name on an official list 登记，注册

(7) abdomen /ˈæbdəmən/ *n.* the part of the body below the chest that contains the stomach, bowels , etc. 腹（部）

(8) intestinal /ɪnˈtestɪnl/ *adj.* 肠的

(9) distention /dɪsˈtenʃən/ *n.* 膨胀，扩张

(10) moxa /ˈmɒksə/ wool 艾绒

(11) ignite /ɪgˈnaɪt/ to start to burn; to make sth. start to burn（使）燃烧

(12) oblique /əˈbliːk/ *adj.* sloping at an angle 倾斜的

(13) malt sugar 麦芽糖

(14) soothe the aches and pains 缓解疼痛

(15) stimulate blood circulation 刺激血液循环

(16) to treat many ailments 治疗病痛

Sentence Patterns

(1) Acupuncture originated in China more than 2,000 years ago. It is one component within the system of traditional Chinese medicine.

(2) Having acupuncture on *Zu San Li* can promote digestion.

(3) Having acupuncture on *Nei Guan* is good for one's heart.

(4) The tiny needles reveal the mysteries of human body.

(5) The major knots on the network are called *Xue Wei*, or an acupuncture point.

(6) TCM doctors believe that stimulating the *Xue Wei* can promote energy circulation and expel illness.

(7) Acupuncture has been practiced for centuries not only in China, but also in Japan, Korea, and Vietnam. The technique spread to Europe about 300 years ago, to North America about 150 years ago, and to countries worldwide within the past 40 years.

(8) The earliest acupuncture tools were sharp pieces of stone or flint, known as *Bianshi* stone.

(9) There are 12 main meridians and 8 secondary meridians. Each of the 12 main meridians is associated with a major internal organ, such as the liver or the heart. According to different practitioners, there are more than 2,000 acupuncture points. Acupuncture needles inserting into these points can unblock and balance the flow of *qi*.

(10) In the United States, the Food and Drug Administration (FDA) approved the use of acupuncture needles by licensed practitioners in 1996. Since then, acupuncture has gained increasing popularity, both used singly or as a complement to Western therapies. Most states have established standards for obtaining acupuncture certification.

(11) The World Health Organization (WHO) lists a wide variety of medical

conditions that may benefit from acupuncture treatment including sciatica, cataracts, bronchitis, insomnia, diarrhea, parkinson disease, and stroke. In addition, research studies suggest that acupuncture may be effective for such conditions as chronic pain, drug and alcohol addiction, migraines, lower back pain, and nausea associated with chemotherapy.

(12) Acupoints are regarded as pathways which run throughout the body to transport life energy.

(13) Acupuncture and moxibustion are highly effective, simple in performance and low in cost, and they have been widely used in China for thousands of years.

(14) Acupuncture and moxibustion can regulate heartbeat, body temperature, blood pressure and respiration, relieve muscle spasm and numbness.

(15) Acupuncture is performed by inserting needles into selected acupuncture points. Typically, a practitioner inserts the needle 3 to 10 mm deep, depending on the condition and treatment objectives. Once inserted, the needles are rotated by hand or are connected to an electrical device that sends low-voltage currents along the needles and into the body. Depending on the patient's condition, needles remain in the body for five minutes to an hour or longer. Some people report feeling energized by an acupuncture treatment, while others feel relaxed.

III Model Dialogues

Conversation 1

Lily: The weight problem has been a nightmare for me. I am so worried about my body shape.

Li Lei: Did you try anything to lose your weight?

Lily: Yes, I tried many ways, such as dieting, diet pill, doing yoga, but all my efforts do not pay off.

Li Lei: Would you like to try acupuncture and moxibustion?

Lily: No. You mean the needles used by doctors of Chinese medicine can help me lose weight. I don't understand how could it be possible.

Li Lei: Well, let me explain the principle of acupuncture for weight loss. Modern medicine has discovered that obesity is mainly caused by endocrine disorder, and acupuncture is effective in regulating endocrine secretion. Besides, Chinese medicine believes that gaining weight is closely related with the function of the spleen, the liver and the kidney, so acupuncture can be used to bring the functions of those *zang*-organs back to normal.

Lily: Sounds good. Does it have any bad effects? I mean, nausea, pain or headache.

Li Lei: Of course not, you will be safe and sound. Trust me. Being painless is one of the edges of acupuncture for weight loss. But you may feel less desire for food, because acupuncture will restrain your eagerness for eating and also the absorption function of your internal organs.

Lily: Which acupoints will doctors prick?

Li Lei: Well, it's complicated. I mean, doctors will diagnose you before deciding which acupoints to prick. But the most commonly used acupoints are *Guan Yuan* which is under the navel and *San Yin Jiao* which is located above the ankle.

Lily: What about moxibustion? Can it also be used to lose weight?

Li Lei: Yes, the principle of moxibustion is actually the same as acupuncture. The only difference is that the former uses the heat giving off by burning moxa stick to stimulate certain acupoints, while the latter uses needles.

Lily: I see. Thank you for your explanation and recommendation. I think I will give it a try.

Conversation 2

Patient: Doctor, I often have abdominal pain. Can it be cured with acupuncture treatment?

Doctor: Yes, of course. Acupuncture is very effective for abdominal pain. Please tell me how you feel when it occurs.

Patient: When it starts, I ache and feel chill all over the abdomen. But when applied with hot pressing and rubbing, the pain would be relieved.

Doctor: Does the situation get worse after you eat cold drinks?

Patient: Yes, once I ate some iced watermelon and the pain nearly killed me.

Doctor: Are your defecation and urine normal?

Patient: The defecation is loose and the urine is clear.

Doctor: Please stick out your tongue. Well, your tongue is pale with white coating. Let me feel your pulse. Er... your pulse is deep and sluggish. Did you take a intestinal check recently?

Patient: Yes, I did it last week, and found nothing abnormal. Doctor, what's wrong with me?

Doctor: In TCM it is abdominal pain due to the insufficiency of kidney yang. I'll apply heat-needling treatment on you. Please lie down.

Patient: Can you tell me what is heat-needling treatment? It sounds scary.

Doctor: Well, don't worry. Heat-needling is a combination of acupuncture and moxibustion applied to the the diseases with the retention of the needles and moxibustion.

Now I'll insert the needle into *Zhong Wan* (RN 12). How do you feel now?

Patient: I feel much distension.

Doctor: This distending feeling is called *De Qi* in TCM, also known as needling sensation. Now you see, I'll cut a piece of moxa wool and attach it to the end of the inserted needle, then ignite the moxa. They can exert a combined effect of acupuncture and heat stimulation. And this is the heat-needling treatment.

Patient: I feel very warm and comfortable.

Doctor: Now, the moxa wool has burned out. Let me pull out the needle. Please turn over, I'll puncture the *Pi Shu* (BL 20) and *Wei Shu* (BL 21) points on the back. By puncturing these two points, as well as *Zhong Wan* (RN 12) point, it can warm the middle energizer to dispel cold and enrich spleen yang.

Patient: Do these two points also need heat-needling?

Doctor: No. Since the skin and muscles of the back are very thin and there are important organs in this part, only oblique insertion can be used. Do you have any sensation?

Patient: Yes. I have the distending sensation.

Doctor: Good. The needles will be retained for 15 minutes. Be sure not to eat anything raw, cold or greasy. But you can eat some Chinese dates and malt sugar. The needling is over. You can stand up now.

Patient: Do I need to take some herbal medicines?

Doctor: Yes. Which do you prefer, drinking the decoction or taking the prepared drugs of herbal medicines?

Patient: Prepared drugs, Please.

Doctor: I'll prescribe 20 pills of *Fuzi Lizhong Wan* for you. You may take one pill twice a day.

Patient: When should I come again?

Doctor: You have to come every morning for the acupuncture treatment.

Patient: All right. Thank you, doctor.

IV Oral Practice

Situational Dialogues

Situation 1

Lily is gaining a lot of weight recently, so she is worrying about her figure. She has tried ways to lose weight, but it seems there is no remarkable effects. Her friend Li Lei is a student majoring in TCM, and he suggests losing weight with the help of Chinese medicine.

Situation 2

Kate looks depressed and worried. Her friend Jim asks her the reason. It is because of Kate's mom who seems suffering from menopausal syndromes. Her mom has tried to see a doctor of Western medicine, but in vain. Jim suggests her mom to try acupuncture of Chinese medicine.

Situation 3

Lee is 30 years old now, and one day when he got up, he found that he had got facial paralysis on the left side of his face. Frightened, he hurried to the hospital to see the doctor who suggested using acupuncture, which is the most effective way to cure Lee's disease. The doctor explains that the function of acupuncture is to expel wind and clear away cold, unblock the channels and regulate the flow of *qi*, since face is the place where the hand-*Yangming Channels* and foot-*Yangming Channels* originate and end, the points of *Yangming Channels* are often chosen. Puncturing the points of *Yang Bai* (GB 14), *Feng Chi* (GB 20) , *Si Bai*(ST 2), *Ying Xiang*(LI 20), *Di Cang*(ST4), *Jia Che*(ST6), *He Gu* (LI4) and applying moxibustion on the point of *Yi Feng* (SJ17)is effective.

Situation 4

The following is a medical record of a patient suffering from chronic diarrhea. The doctor describes the information about the patient and treatment process in the medical record. Please make up a dialogue based on the following case.

A Case of Chronic Diarrhea

Info.of the Patient

Female, 45 years, American

The patient has developed obesity, diarrhea with fatigue for more than 10 years since her first childbirth. She was diagnosed with diverticulosis by a local doctor, and she tried some therapies including anti-biotics, supplements and acupuncture, but without any improvement. Recently, she usually has diarrhea for 6-10 times per day, the stool was in dark color, water-like, often accompanied with mild abdominal pain, denied any blood or mucus in her stool. Sometimes, the patient may feel a sensation of cold and dampness inside her abdomen. She prefers warm water and liquid diet, and always feels fatigue. Denied abnormal sweating. Her sleep was normal, sometimes she has burning sensation in her lower abdomen during urination.

The patient has done surgeries for appendicitis and tonsillitis since she was young. Denied other history of chronic diseases, communicable diseases. Denied any specified food and medicine allergy. But she's intolerant to dairy product and rice.

Her menstruation was on time but with decreased volume and loose.The patient is a social smoker. Denied any history of alcohol abuse.

On Inspection: enlarged pale tongue, thick yellowish greasy coating, sinking slippery pulse, weak in her right hand.

Diagnosis: Diverticulitis, obesity, diarrhea disorder.

Pattern: Yang deficiency of spleen and kidney with dampness retention in middle energizer.

Therapeutic principle: Enhancing yang of both spleen and kidney, and expelling dampness.

Treatment with Acupuncture: Right *Xue Hai* (SP10), *Yin Ling Quan* (SP9), left *Zu San Li* (ST36), *San Yin Jiao* (SP6).

Moxibustion: *Shen Que* (CV8), *Guan Yuan* (CV4), both *Zu San Li* (ST36), *Yin Ling Quan* (SP9).

Suggestions: change habit of diet, avoid cold and raw food, try soup of lotus seeds, yam and job's tears with sliced fresh ginger or ginger juice.

At the end of one session, as diarrhea vanished, the patient regained her appetite though still suffering from weight loss by 1 kg. The following therapies for the patient lasted for more than one month. Dr Wang reduced the use of acupuncture and tried to enhance yang *qi* in her spleen and kidney with moxibustion. No relapse of diarrhea was found. And her fatigue faded away.

Chronic diarrhea is consumptive when patients are losing body fluid every day, in the mean time, they're also losing *qi*, because body fluid is the carrier of *qi*. When the body is lacking of *qi*, the loss of body fluid may get worse, because the flow of body fluid is normally governed by *qi*. A vicious circle may be formed so that enhancing *qi* is a good way to break this circle. Moxibustion works quite well in enhancing yangqi by securing blood and body fluids if it's been properly used. The patient responds quite well to our therapy. According to Dr Wang, of course, it is not the end of the treatment. But unfortunately, it is the end of the story.

"It feels like constipation when I suddenly have stool once a day. And it took me one week to get used to normal stool. Thank you very much," said the patient.

Story Retelling

Cue Words

(1) 炼丹   make pills of immortality/ to make elixir

(2) 行医   to practice medicine/ to work as doctors

(3) 针灸师   acupuncturist

(4) 瘤   tumor

(5) 疣   wart

(6) 艾   moxa, wormwood

(7) 红脚艾   red-feet wormwood

(8)《肘后备急方》 *Handbook of Prescriptions for Emergencies*

鲍姑是中国晋代著名的女医生。她与丈夫葛洪在广东罗浮山炼丹行医，当地人民尊称她为"鲍仙姑"。鲍姑尤其精通灸法，是中国医学史上第一位女针灸学家。

鲍姑治疗赘瘤和赘疣特别出名。为治好这种病，她总结了以前人们治病的经验，就地取材，采用越秀山上的红脚艾进行灸疗。用这种艾灸治人身上的赘瘤，一灼就消，疗效非常好，因此，后人称之为"鲍姑艾"。据说经过鲍姑灸疗的病人，不仅身上的赘瘤和赘疣能立刻消除，而且不留疤痕，容颜也变得更加美丽。

很遗憾，鲍姑没有留下什么著作，她的灸法经验可能留在葛洪的《肘后备急方》中了。这本书有灸方九十余条，对灸法的作用、效果、操作方法、注意事项等都有较全面的论述。

Group Task

The Magical Function of Acupuncture

On Wikipedia, acupuncture is regarded as a pseudoscience. However, the truth is that acupuncture has been widely used in China for over 2000 years, and currently it has been recognized in countries, such as America, Australia, and some European countries. It is widely practiced in China, and one of the most common alternative medicine practices in Europe. In 2010, UNESCO inscribed "acupuncture of traditional Chinese medicine" on the UNESCO Intangible Cultural Heritage List following China's nomination.

In the summer of 1971, James Reston, then vice president of *The New York Times*, visited China at the invitation of the Chinese government. During the period, due to acute appendicitis, Reston was admitted to Peking Union Medical College Hospital and underwent appendectomy. On the second day after the operation, Reston developed abdominal distension and pain. Chinese doctors treated him with acupuncture.

According to Reston, a young Chinese acupuncturist put three needles under his right elbow and knees, and seared his abdomen with a "cheap cigar like" moxa roll, which significantly reduced his abdominal distension.

Later, James Reston published a report on the front page of *The New York Times* entitled "*Now, About My Operation In Peking*". It was only after that acupuncture therapy began to receive widespread attention from European and American countries.

In 2003 WHO reported that acupuncture had been proved to be effective for more than a hundred kinds of diseases.

In 2020, *Shanghai Daily* published a news report titled "*Acupuncture Helping Coronavirus Patients*". Medical workers from Yueyang Hospital of Integrated traditional Chinese and Western medicine have been giving novel coronavirus disease patients at Wuhan's *Leishenshan* Hospital acupuncture, an effective treatment for those with problems such as insomnia and migraines.

"Traditional Chinese medicine plays an important role in treating patients during the outbreak of coronavirus disease. It tells us that traditional Chinese medicine, the treasure of our country, should never be abandoned and we should pay more attention to it for its better development and inheritance."

What's more, acupuncture is found to be effective for relieving pain for women. Researchers in Australia and New Zealand have found that acupuncture can significantly reduce the severity and duration of period pain. The study conducted by Australian and New Zealand researchers also found it relieved associated headaches and nausea.

There are more for you to explore about the use of acupuncture.

Oral Task

Please prepare a report introducing the development of acupuncture, including some important events related with acupuncture, such as the inventions of acupuncture anesthesia and the founding of World Federation of Acupuncture-Moxibustion Societies（世界针灸学会联合会）. You should also include the analysis of the drawbacks of acupuncture and suggestions for its better development in your report.

Reading and Question Answering

Acupuncture Treats Post-COVID Conditions Overseas

TCM puts patients in United States on road to recovery.

When Elvira Figueroa, a 69-year-old hairdresser in New York, found she had COVID-19 in March last year, she thought she was going to die.

"I got every symptom you can imagine," she said. "First, I had a horrible headache for two days, then I started a high fever. Then it went to my lungs. I lost 25 pounds (11.33 kilograms). I was so sick that I didn't remember many things."

After Figueroa recovered, she began to experience post-COVID-19 conditions, or long COVID—a term that refers to symptoms that linger for weeks or months beyond infection.

"I had no energy and I was very weak. I was constantly exhausted. I took vitamin E and vitamin C, as my cardiologist advised. I had to retire. My nails were getting black, my feet were bleeding. So many things were wrong," she said.

Her cardiologist recommended that she try acupuncture. "It helped me tremendously. I was very, very happy," Figueroa said.

She added that acupuncture helped relieve bodily inflammation and eased pain in her back.

Treatment for post-COVID-19 conditions among many people in the United States now involves lying in a room with warm lighting, listening to relaxing music and watching dozens of needles inserted into one's body.

Practiced in China for thousands of years, acupuncture traditionally involves inserting thin metal needles into specific points in the ears or other parts of the body to relieve pain and restore energy flow.

Studies have shown that COVID-19 causes what is known as a cytokine storm, leading to inflammation that could kill tissue and damage organs. Last year, a study by Harvard University found that acupuncture reduced the impact of cytokine storms in mice.

The Harvard researchers also found that animals treated with acupuncture immediately before they developed a cytokine storm experienced lower levels of inflammation during subsequent disease and fared better than those that were not treated.

Chinese experts found that acupuncture treatment for COVID-19 suppressed inflammation caused by stress, improved immunity, regulated nervous system functions and helped cancer patients with COVID.

Help for the body

Kai Zhang, a doctor from Tianjin Gong An Hospital, said, "Acupuncture cannot kill the virus directly, but it can regulate the immune system and inhibit inflammation, helping the body fight the virus."

The *Wall Street Journal* reported that an estimated 10 percent to 30 percent of COVID-19 patients have symptoms weeks and months after first becoming ill, including many young, previously healthy people who initially had mild cases of the disease.

According to the US Centers for Disease Control and Prevention, the most common lasting symptoms are fatigue, shortness of breath, coughing, joint pain and chest pain. Other issues include cognitive problems, difficulty concentrating, depression, muscle pain, headaches, rapid heartbeat and intermittent fever.

New York resident Naoko Baynes said that after having acupuncture, her life returned to normal. She had dysosmia—a disorder that affects the sense of smell—for a year. Infected with the coronavirus in March last year, she was only able to smell burning tires and rotten bananas when she recovered.

"I tried smell training—using four essential oils twice a day for 10 minutes. The oils are meant to cover the four groups of smell. I did this for months and nothing changed," she said. "I didn't try acupuncture until December. They started by putting needles in my face near my nose and also in my wrists and the crook of the elbow. It was painful, but once the needles were in and twisted, it was fine."

"I felt no change, but then my senses of smell and taste had major shifts over the course of six months, and now I'm 90 percent back to normal. I still have some difficulty with very delicate smells, but that is also changing," she said.

Jasmine Hong Lai, a licensed acupuncturist and certified herbalist in New York State, said acupuncture is "pretty good" for treating post-COVID conditions such as coughs, changes in smell or taste, fatigue and headaches.

According to the Kaiser Family Foundation, a nonprofit organization based in San Francisco, about four in ten US adults have reported symptoms of anxiety or depression during the pandemic, a level that has been largely consistent. Such symptoms were reported by one in ten adults from January to June 2019.

In June, Lai started to treat patients with post-COVID conditions. Most of them were experiencing fatigue and headaches.

When Samantha Scher, a 27-year-old lawyer, recovered from COVID-19, she experienced fainting, severe headaches and dizziness.

"When I started acupuncture, my body was so bad as a result of COVID and the medicine the hospital gave me when I kept fainting. I felt very tired and nauseous," she said.

After Scher tried acupuncture for a month, she started to feel she was returning to normal.

"I had not had acupuncture before, until COVID. I was afraid of needles, and I had to close my eyes. But as I had very bad anxiety and depression at that time, I didn't really care about the needles. I just needed anything to help," Scher said.

This year marks the 50th anniversary of the broad use of acupuncture in the US. In 1971, *The New York Times* columnist James Reston opened the door for the treatment in the US. When Reston traveled to China as part of the advance team before US President Richard Nixon's visit the following year, he had an acute attack of appendicitis. While Reston was hospitalized in China, his pain was treated with acupuncture.

He wrote of his experiences with Chinese medicine, and the reports he filed, along with his observations on the effectiveness of acupuncture, helped pave the way for the exploration of alternative medicine in the US.

Insurance cover

Last year, Medicare, the largest US federal government insurance program, began covering acupuncture as a treatment for lower back pain due to the nation's opioid crisis. Medicare covers up to 12 sessions in 90 days, with an additional eight sessions for patients with chronic lower back pain who show improvement.

Lai said: "In the US, many people recognize the effect of acupuncture in the treatment of pain, but acupuncture is also very good at treating indigestion, gynecological issues like infertility, and mental issues such as insomnia, anxiety and depression. The good thing is that more people are gaining knowledge of acupuncture."

In the US, an acupuncturist needs to complete an accredited educational program and pass a state licensing exam.

Su, the New York and Connecticut acupuncturist, said: "Some acupuncturists graduated from Chinese medicine universities in China, some of them graduated from colleges of traditional Chinese medicine in the US. As long as you meet the assessments designed by the National Certification Commission for Acupuncture and Oriental Medicine and the state licensing exam, you can become an acupuncturist."

According to the American Institution of Alternative Medicine, a bachelor's degree in acupuncture is needed to qualify as a practitioner. The degree takes four years to complete if studying full-time.

Acupuncture Today reported that some 50 schools and colleges in the US provide education in acupuncture and Chinese medicine, and they receive thousands of students every year.

Oral Tasks

Prepare a 2-minute report about the use of acupuncture in China.

You should say:

The diseases which can be treated with acupuncture;

How do patients generally feel about acupuncture;

Your personal views on acupuncture.

V Creative Oral Activity

Re Min Jiu (Heat-sensitive Moxibustion)

Originated from *Nei Jing* (*Yellow Emperor's Canon of Medicine*), thermosensitive moxibustion, also known as heat-sensitive moxibustion is a patent technology invented by professor Chen Rixin of Jiangxi Provincial Hospital of Chinese Medicine. Heat-sensitive moxibustion is a treatment using the burning moxa stick to stimulate heat-sensitive acupoints. It features zero contact with the human body, harm free, and no side effects.

Upon receiving *Re Min Jiu* treatment, one may feel the heat penetrating, expanding, moving over the surface of body. Someone may fail to feel the heat, which can also be called heat sensitivity. In 2010, achievements of *Re Min Jiu* was firstly displayed in Shanghai EXPO. The first *Re Min Jiu* hospital in the world was established in 2011 in Nanchang, Jiangxi province. Because of its outstanding clinical effects, *Re Min Jiu* has been spread at home and even abroad.

Professor Chen and his team have made researches on 6 kinds of diseases, 360 heat-sensitive acupoints and found that distribution of the heat sensitivity of the acupoints is a dynamic process and surrounded by the meridian acupoints according to the disease change.

The meridian *qi* can be stimulated by moxibustion on the heat-sensitive acupoints, and can be transmitted to affected areas, thus producing highly curative effect. The incidence rate of stimulating and transmitting meridian *qi* to the disease area by moxibustion on heat-sensitive acupoints is 86.73%, while that by moxibustion on non-heatsensitive acupoints is only 22.41%.

Up till now, it has been proved that heat-sensitive moxibustion can be used to effectively treat diseases like joint pain, joint deformity and hypertension.

Oral Task

Activity 1

Suppose you are a doctor on *Re Min Jiu* and a foreigner goes to see you for treatment. Please make up a dialogue based on the given situation.

Activity 2

Please search for more information on *Re Min Jiu*, and then make a brief report on it.

Chapter Eleven

Sub-health and Health Preservation

Learning Objectives

In this chapter you will learn:

● How to describe sub-health, namely its causes, manifestations, and solutions;

● Conversational expressions and skills on sub-healthy conditions.

I Lead-in Questions

(1) How healthy do you think you are?

(2) Do you ever feel psychological fatigue?

(3) Do you lead a healthy or unhealthy life style? Why?

(4) What do you usually do to keep healthy?

(5) Which is more terrible, getting sick or sub-healthy?

II Useful Expressions

New Words and Phrases

(1) nutritious /njuˈtrɪʃəs/ *adj.* of or providing nourishment 有营养的，滋养的

(2) sub-health /sʌb helθ/ *n.* 亚健康

(3) fatigue /fəˈtiːg/ *n.* temporary loss of strength and energy resulting from hard physical or mental work 疲劳，疲乏

(4) relieve /rɪˈliːv/ *vt.* provide physical relief, as from pain 解除，减轻

(5) acupoint /ˈækjʊpɒɪnt/ *n.* 穴道，穴位

(6) massage /ˈmæsɑːʒ/ *v.* manually manipulate (someone's body), usually for medicinal or relaxation purposes 按摩

(7) constipation /ˌkɒnstɪˈpeɪʃn/ *n.* irregular and infrequent or difficult evacuation of the bowels 便秘

(8) sluggish /ˈslʌgɪʃ/ *adj.* with little movement; very slow 萧条的，迟钝的

(9) agitate /ˈædʒɪteɪt/ *vt.* cause to be agitated, excited, or roused 使…激动

(10) fragile /ˈfrædʒaɪl/ *adj.* easily broken or damaged or destroyed 脆的，易碎的

(11) prone /prəʊn/ *adj.* having a tendency (to) 易于…的

(12) insomnia /ɪnˈsɒmniə/ *n.* someone who suffers from insomnia finds it difficult to sleep 失眠症，失眠

(13) appetite /ˈæpɪtaɪt/ *n.* a feeling of craving something 食欲

(14) inspection /ɪnˈspekʃn/ *n.* a formal or official examination 检查

(15) eliminate /ɪˈlɪmɪneɪt/ *vt.* terminate or take out 消除，排除

(16) contamination /kənˌtæmɪˈneɪʃn/ *n.* the state of being contaminated 污染，玷污

(17) excessive /ɪkˈsesɪv/ *adj.* beyond normal limits 过多的，极度的

(18) priority /praɪˈɒrəti/ *n.* status established in order of importance or urgency 优先，优先权

(19) transgenic /ˌtrænzˈdʒenɪk; ˌtrænsˈdʒenɪk/ *adj.* 转基因的，基因改造的

(20) preservative /prɪˈzɜːvətɪv/ *n.* a chemical compound that is added to protect against decay or decomposition 防腐剂

Sentence Patterns

How to introduce sub-health and its damage

(1) Sub-health, also called the third state, is a gray period between healthy conditions and disease or unhealthy conditions.

(2) According to a recent survey, sub-health is afflicting 60% of the middle-aged and elderly.

(3) Females are more susceptible to sub-health than males.

(4) Sub-health has already been considered as the new killer of human health.

(5) The characteristic of sub-health is that it occurs between the ages of 20 and 50, and is more prevalent among people with higher educational level.

(6) The main syndromes for sub-health are manifested by bodily fatigue, difficulty in recovering after rest, body-ache, dizziness with headache, sleep disorders, lack of appetite, insomnia, dreaminess, palpitation, depression, anxiety, stress, fear, bad temper, and unsociable and eccentric behavior.

(7) Some serious patients suffer from low self-esteem with no desire for progress, loss of memory and concentration, and low efficiency in work and study.

(8) In contemporary society, the quickening pace of life in modern society has put

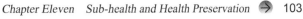

some in the working class at a state of over-strain.

(9) According to traditional Chinese medicine, sub-health is caused by many reasons which connect with modern lifestyle like rapid life pace, fierce competition, strong pressure, bad habits and environmental pollution.

(10) Sub-health is reflected by the disorders of organic functions and irritable moody state.

(11) Office workers are the major victims of sub-health, including high-tech personnel, senior intellectuals, medical treatment personnel, IT staff, traffic police, etc.

(12) The condition of Chinese white-collar workers in the mainland has received a bad prognosis with 60 percent over fatigued and 76 percent in sub-health.

(13) Congenital deficiency, bad living habits or being stimulated by character, the pressure from the fast speed of life and work, environmental pollution and unfavorable weather can cause sub-health.

(14) Keeping a good mood, having proper exercise and regulating our diet and living habits could help alleviate the symptoms of sub-health.

How to stay healthy in daily life based on TCM

(1) The first way is to balance the nutrition, which is the base of health. Any kind of food can not provide certain nutrients the body needs.

(2) To ensure adequate sleep is the second way to improve sub-health. There is a close relationship between sleep and human health.

(3) People should keep proper balance between work and rest, be optimistic even facing with troubles in life and learn to adjust to the geographical and climatic changes.

(4) Staying healthy via TCM has become popular in recent years.

(5) Appropriate and continuous exercises can promote the flow of *qi* and blood, which can improve digestion and blood circulation, and enhance immune system.

(6) *Taichi* is an traditional aerobic exercise for stress reduction and health improvement.

(7) Wise men always emphasize disease prevention before its occurrence.

III Model Dialogues

Conversation 1

Li Ming: Hi, Lily. I don't mean to disturb you, but you truly don't look very well. What's the matter with you?

Lily: Oh, thank you, Li Ming. You are so nice. I don't know what is wrong with me.

I slept badly recently, you know, I find it difficult to fall asleep at night. And I slept only a few hours every night.

Li Ming: I am sorry to hear that. You see, I know something about Chinese medicine. Maybe I can be of some help to you.

Lily: Really! That's the best news I've heard recently. Thank you, Li Ming.

Li Ming: How long have you been like this?

Lily: It's been quite a while, two months or so.

Li Ming: Do you have any other symptoms besides insomnia?

Lily: Yes, I feel shortness of breath. And I don't feel like eating at all. And sometimes, I have severe headache which seems to crack my head into two halves.

Li Ming: Are you under any stress recently?

Lily: Yes, I guess so. I have been writing my thesis in the past two months, and it is not going smoothly. I stay up late nearly every night in order to write the thesis, and I will soon finish it.

Li Ming: If you do not mind, I want to know whether you have any diseases?

Lily: No, I seldom get sick.

Li Ming: Well, I guess I have found the cause for your problem. Stress is to blame. When you finish your thesis, you should sleep early to make up what you have lost, and relax by travelling somewhere, I guess you'll be sound and healthy again. And you can press the Bai Hui acupoint with your thumb for two to three minutes a day, which can relieve your pain.

Lily: Thank you, Li Ming. I feel much better now.

Conversation 2

Jack: Hi, Li Ming. I read an alarming report yesterday that about 70% of the population in China are under the sub-health state. Well, that is not unexpected. Due to the fast-paced life style, more and more people have ignored the importance of healthy diet and sleeping.

Li Ming: As you know, sub-health is the boundary state between health and illness, so it is truly a worrisome issue. What's worse, people who are under this state are more likely to get cancer, especially liver cancer, so sub-health is regarded as the No.1 enemy to people's health in the 21st century.

Jack: I am so worried that I may be in sub-health condition.

Li Ming: Come on, my friend. You are still young, so there is fat chance you get sub-health.

Jack: No, you don't understand. Recently, I notice that I have a lot of health problems, such as hair loss, short of breath, loss of concentration, and I can easily get angry over some trivial things.

Li Ming: Maybe, it is because you are too tired. I know you are busy preparing for an important test.

Jack: Yes, I have been preparing for the test for 3 months. But before that I have kept the bad habit of sleeping late hours for many years, and I often eat junk food. So I guess it's the long-time bad habit that finally does damage to my health.

Li Ming: Did you go to the hospital for body checking?

Jack: Yes, I did it last week, but the physical examination showed that I had nothing wrong.

Li Ming: Don't worry. You can try Chinese medicine which is very effective to improve the state of sub-health. "Prevention before the onset of diseases" is an important concept of health preservation in Chinese medicine.

Jack: Sounds good. Then what should I do?

Li Ming: Well, there are many ways to improve your health state in Chinese medicine, but I like drinking herbal tea to strengthen the functions of internal organs and unblock channels.

Jack: Really? How is the effect?

Li Ming: Well, I have been drinking a tea called *Yujin Guiyuan Tea* for several months. It contains some herbal medicines like longan and American ginseng and can nourish the blood and *yin*. After drinking the tea, I feel that I am full of energy and I don't get sick any more.

Jack: Amazing! I will try the magical Chinese herbal tea.

Li Ming: I have a good doctor of Chinese medicine to recommend for you, and I guess he will offer you some professional help.

Jack: Thank you, Li Ming.

IV Oral Practice

Situational Dialogues

Work in teams and make up dialogues based on the following situations.

Situation 1

Suppose you are a student majoring in TCM and one of your relatives has been suffering from sub-health. Make a phone call to him/her and give some advice on keeping physical and mental health.

Situation 2

You are a student majoring in TCM. Your friend Jack is asking you about how to maintain health. You give him some tips as follows.

(1) Massage "*Zu San Li*" and "*Yong Quan*" in daily life, because those two acupoints are called "acupoints of longevity" . Pressing "*Zu San Li*" can improve the digestive function of the stomach, while pressing "*Yong Quan*" is good for strengthening the back and waist, so it is beneficial for old people.

(2) Combing hair. It is both a convenient and cheap way of keeping fit. When we are combing hair, we are stimulating the acupoints and meridians on the head, so it can ensure the free flow of blood and *qi* on head, thus further regulating the circulation of blood and *qi* all over the body. And it can relieve headache, loss of hair and vertigo.

(3) Food therapy. Eat healthy and balanced diet including fruits and vegetables but less meat.

Situation 3

Have a discussion with your partner(s).

Here is an example of a daily health-care proposal.

Five "A"

A smile everyday;

An hour's exercise everyday;

A cup of warm water in the morning;

A fruit everyday;

A cup of milk before sleep.

Story Retelling

Cue Words

(1) 铁锅　iron pot

(2) 肥胖症　obesity

(3) 两　liang, a unit of weight (=50 grams)

(4) 瓜子　sunflower seeds

(5) 里　li, a unit of length (=500 meters)

巧治肥胖症

东汉时期，华佗在路上见到一个胖子，他的肚子大得像口大铁锅，正气喘吁吁地往前走。华佗说："我是医生，我给你治治这肥胖症吧。"

　　华佗问了他的饮食起居习惯，然后说："你每天准备二两瓜子，天一亮就起床，一边吃瓜子一边走路，把瓜子吃完后再按照原路走回来，中间不许休息。三个月后就能见效。"只吃瓜子、走路就能减肥，胖子心想这真是好事，于是他回家后第二天一大早就照着做了，一直走了五里多路才把瓜子吃完，然后又按原路走回家。开始几天，他累得满身大汗，两条腿重得走不动，但中间又不敢休息。就这样十多天过去了，他渐渐觉得腿不那么重了，汗也出得少了，浑身也有力气了。三个月后，身上果然少了很多肉，连大肚子也没有了。

　　为了表示感谢，胖子去看望华佗。华佗告诉他："从现在开始，要早睡早起，多干点活，多吃青菜，少吃肉，这样能完全治好你的肥胖症。"胖子听完，高高兴兴地回家去了。

Group Task

An increasingly large number of people are suffering from sub-health nowadays. According to TCM, sub-health is caused by many reasons which are closely related with modern lifestyle, like rapid life pace, severe competition, pressure, improper living habits and environmental pollution. Sub-health is reflected by the disorders of physiological functions and irritable moody state. In order to keep healthy, it is necessary for people to alleviate and avoid sub-health. Work with your partners and finish the following group task:

● What are the signs of a person being in the state of sub-health?

● In *Huangdi's Internal Classic*, it holds that "A superior doctor treat the disease before its onset." (上工治未病), "The sages usually pay less attention to the treatment of a disease, but more to the prevention of it." (圣人不治已病治未病) "The sages cultivate yang in spring and summer while nourish yin in autumn and winter." (圣人春夏养阳，秋冬养阴). What do you think is the proper way to keep healthy, especially with the help of TCM? Work in groups and present your oral report in PPT.

Reading and Question Answering

A health report on Shanghai white-collar workers became a trending topic on China's Twitter-like Sina Weibo on Wednesday with it showing that, for Shanghai's office workers, the abnormal rate of physical examinations has astonishingly risen to nearly 99 percent, with fewer than two in every 100 office workers "completely healthy" .

Chinese workers' "poor" health condition and tech companies' toxic "996" work culture —which involves working from 9 am to 9 pm six days a week—have made waves in Chinese people's online discourse since the first workday of 2021 following the sudden death of a 23-year-old employee at China's e-commerce giant Pinduoduo, believed to be related to her overworking until 1:30 am on December 29, 2020.

Many netizens advocated the local authorities to prohibit working overtime because many workers have faced overworking.

One netizen commented that it is hard to say whether the current generation can expect to live longer than previous generations even with today's advanced medical science techniques, because many incurable diseases still exist, and postponing retirement will only make the situation worse.

According to the 2019 Report on Shanghai White-collar Workers' Health Index jointly released by Shanghai Foreign Service (Group) Co. (FSG) and the Popular Medicine magazine, the abnormal rate of physical examinations for Shanghai's office workers rose to 98.75 percent in 2018 from 94 percent in 2013.

In terms of genders, the top three health problems for women include bone rarefaction, helicobacter pylori and chronic cervicitis, while the top three problems for men were increased blood viscosity, thyroid disorders and chronic pharyngitis.

Research conducted by the FSG shows that unhealthy habits, such as staying up late, psychological pressure (mainly from work), and lack of exercise have become the major factors affecting white-collar workers' health in Shanghai.

It is noteworthy that the youngest generation of the workforce who were born in the 1990s have also suffered from health issues such as skin problems, anxiety and depression, and intestine and stomach problems, according to a report on Chinese nationals' health released by DXY.com in 2019.

A health consultant surnamed Cao at a local physical checkup center in Shanghai told the Global Times on Wednesday that according to her over 40 years' medical treatment experience in internal medicine, she advised office workers to pay attention to their annual physical checkup and advocated for early detection and treatment of diseases.

"The fundamental problem that causes people's sub-health problems and diseases is the lack of a regular work and rest schedule and unadjusted psychological problems, which stands out as a social problem," said Cao, who noted that unsolved psychological problems ultimately manifest themselves through physical illnesses.

Questions

(1) Why is there a higher chance for office workers to suffer from sub-health?

(2) What is your suggestion for young people to get rid of sub-health by means of Chinese medicine?

V Creative Oral Activity

Task 1

A group of foreign guests are now visiting the Jiangzhong Pharmacy (江中制药), and you work as a guide to show them around. Those visitors show great interest in the product of monkey head mushroom biscuit. Please read the introduction of monkey head mushroom as provided below and then introduce the medical snack to the visitors.

Introduction to monkey head mushroom

In China, monkey head mushroom, together with bear paw, shark fin and sea cucumber are regarded as "The Four Famous Dishes". Monkey head mushroom is not only a delicious dish, but also used as a medicinal raw material. In Qing Dynasty, it served as a tribute to the royal family. As for its medicinal value, it has the function of nourishing the stomach and treating stomach illnesses such as duodenal ulcer and CG (Chronic Gastritis) .

Task 2

Everybody has the potential and dream to create something new, and creation is the driving force for the development of science and technology. Many hi-tech products originate from people's inspiration, such as Dajiang UAVs, and isn't it a creation to combine biscuit and stomach nourishment and create a monkey head mushroom biscuit? What do you want to create, especially in your research field? Share it with us.

Chapter Twelve

Chinese Herbal Medicine

....

> **Learning Objectives**
>
> In this chapter you will learn:
> - The properties and actions of Chinese herbs;
> - Instructions of decocting Chinese herbal medicine;
> - Different forms of herbal formulas;
> - A series of conversational expressions on Chinese herbal medicines.

I　Lead-in Questions

(1) What kind of herbs have you ever used?

(2) How do you think about Chinese herbs compared with Western medicine?

(3) What herbs can you find in your living environment? Name some of them.

(4) What are some of the most popular medicinal herbs in China?

(5) Do you know any herbs and their medical functions?

II　Useful Expressions

New Words and Phrases

(1) therapeutic /ˌθerəˈpjuːtɪk/ *adj.* tending to cure or restore to health 治疗的

(2) toxicity /tɒkˈsɪsəti/ *n.* the degree to which something is poisonous 毒性

(3) mutual /ˈmjuːtʃuə/ *adj.* common to or shared by two or more parties 相互的

(4) inhibition /ˌɪnhɪˈbɪʃn/ *n.* the process whereby nerves can retard or prevent the functioning of an organ or part 抑制

(5) antagonism /ænˈtægənɪzəm/ *n.* the relation between opposing principles or forces or factors 对抗，敌对

(6) prescription /prɪˈskrɪpʃn/ *n.* a drug that is available only with written instructions from a doctor or dentist to a pharmacist 药方

(7) constitution /ˌkɒnstɪˈtjuːʃn/ *n.* the way in which someone or something is composed 体格

(8) formula /ˈfɔːmjələ/ *n.* directions for making something 配方

(9) administer /ədˈmɪnɪstə(r)/ *vt.* give or apply (medications）服药

(10) dosage/ˈdəʊsɪdʒ/ *n.* the quantity of an active agent (substance or radiation) taken in or absorbed at any one time 剂量，用量

(11) solution /səˈluːʃn/ *n.* a homogeneous mixture of two or more substances; frequently (but not necessarily) a liquid solution 溶液

(12) tablet /ˈtæblət/ *n.* a dose of medicine in the form of a small pellet 药片

(13) capsule /ˈkæpsjuːl/ *n.* a pill in the form of a small rounded gelatinous container with medicine inside 胶囊

(14) syndrome /ˈsɪndrəʊm/ *n.* a pattern of symptoms indicative of some disease 综合症状

(15) acrid /ˈækrɪd/ *adj.* strong and sharp 辛辣的，苦的

(16) decoction /dɪˈkɒkʃn/ *n.* the extraction of the water-soluble substances of a drug or medicinal plants by boiling 药汤

(17) invigorate /ɪnˈvɪ g əreɪt/ *vt.* give life or energy to 使精力充沛

(18) efficacy /ˈefɪkəsi/ *n.* capacity or power to produce a desired effect 功效，效力

(19) expiry /ɪkˈspaɪəri/ date 过期日期

(20) precipitate /prɪˈsɪpɪteɪt/ *v.* separate as a fine suspension of solid particles 使沉淀

(21) dispel /dɪˈspel/ *vt.* force to go away 驱散，消除

(22) composition /ˌkɒmpəˈzɪʃn/ *n.* 成分

(23) regulate menstruation /ˌmenstruˈeɪʃn/ 调理月经

(24) relieve pain 镇痛

(25) moistening intestine 润肠

(26) side-effect 副作用

(27) adverse effect 不良反应

(28) storage method 贮存方法

(29) instruction（服用）说明

(30) toxic ingredient 有毒成分

(31) nutritional and medicinal effects 营养和药用效果

(32) Chinese patent medicine 中成药

(33) four properties（四气）: cold, hot, warm and cool

(34) five flavors（五味）: acrid/ pungent, sweet, sour, bitter and salty

Sentence Patterns

(1) Chinese medicine is the crystallization of human wisdom.

(2) Chinese herbs refer to medicines used in the prevention, treatment, diagnosis of diseases, rehabilitation therapy, and health care functions under the guidance of traditional Chinese medicine theory.

(3) It contains botanical medicine made from roots, stems, leaves, and fruits of plants, animal medicine made from viscera, skin, and bone of animals, and mineral medicine made from ores.

(4) Chinese herbs need to be correctly used to improve people's health.

(5) Some Chinese herbs need to be made into herbal tea and decoction. Some Chinese herbs need to be ground into a powder to make pellets, ointments, and medicinal liquor.

(6) Chinese herbs are usually used singly or in compound.

(7) There are different categories of Chinese herbs, such as the whole plant, leaf, flower, pollen, fruit, seed, root, rhizome, tree buck, root buck, etc.

(8) Purposes of herbal processing is to improve therapeutic effects, reduce toxicity, drastic properties and side effects, modify properties and actions, and facilitate decocting.

(9) Methods of processing are various, such as discarding impurity, breaking into fine pieces and cutting, rinsing, washing, soaking, splashing, power-refining method with water, parching, stir-frying with liquid, burning, calcining, roasting in hot ashes, steaming, boiling, blanching, stewing, fermentation and germination.

(10) There are four moving directions of Chinese herbs, namely ascending, floating, sinking, and descending.

(11) There are seven kinds of relations as to medicinal compatibility: single application, mutual reinforcement, mutual resistance, mutual assistance, mutual restraint, mutual suppression, mutual inhibition, antagonism.

(12) There are different forms of herbal formulas, such as decoction, pills, powders, pastes, pellets, wine preparation, distillate, suppository, syrup and injection.

(13) The functions of medicinal herbs are exterior-releasing, heat-clearing, downward-draining or precipitating, wind-damp-dispelling and orifice-opening.

III Model Dialogues

Conversation 1

Li Ming: Thank you for dropping by, sit down please. I will brew some dampness-dispelling tea for you.

Jack: Sounds great. I guess I have too much dampness in my body.

Li Ming: How do you know you are having dampness in your body?

Jack: Well, I consulted a doctor of Chinese medicine last week, and I told the doctor that my tongue coating was whitish and thick, my face was always oily, and I often have severe pain in my joints. Anyway, the doctor said that I just had all the symptoms of dampness.

Li Ming: Then you must be extra careful, my friend. I will recommend a formula for you. Give me a minute to prepare all the ingredients.

Jack: I can recognize some of these herbal medicines. These are wolfberry, jujube date and Fuling. I use them for congee. But I don't know the black peel and the thing that looks like rice.

Li Ming: Well, they are preserved tangerine peel and coix seed.

Jack: What is the function of this formula? To dispel dampness?

Li Ming: Well, more than that. The tangerine peel and Fulin help to strengthen the spleen and dispel dampness. Wolfberry serves to tonify the liver and the kidney. Jujube date can supplement *qi* and nourish the blood. And coix seed can improve urination and relieve swelling.

Jack: Wow, this is indeed a miracle formula. Chinese medicine is truly amazing.

Li Ming: It's done. Come on, have a sip. How do you like it?

Jack: En, it not only looks beautiful, but also tastes good. A little bit sweet.

Li Ming: But remember you won't get instant effect after drinking the tea. It will take a long time before you see the effect.

Jack: I know. I will continue to drink the tea everyday. Thank you for your tea.

Conversation 2

Patient: Good morning, doctor. Nice to see you again. Any impression on me?

Doctor: Of course, Mr. Wang. So why are you here again?

Patient: Well, here is the thing. You prescribed a Chinese herbal formula to me, and I went away immediately, but I forgot to ask you how to decoct the medicine. Can you give me some instructions?

Doctor: Sorry, it is my fault. There were too many patients yesterday, so I forgot.

Patient: It doesn't matter.

Doctor: Well, you need to soak the medicine I prescribed to you in water for 15 minutes before you boil them.

Patient: What kind of utensils should I use to boil the medicine.

Doctor: Pottery or ceramic pots with lids. Don't use metal pot, because the medicine may react with metal utensil and harmful elements may be produced during the process.

Patient: Ok, I will bear that in mind.

Patient: What about water? Can I use running water or should I use bottled water?

Doctor: Well, that doesn't matter too much. But spring water might be better.

Patient: Then any matters need attention when I am boiling the medicine?

Doctor: Well, for each package of medicine, you need to use 900mL water. First you use big fire to boil the water, then turn the fire into simmer mode for two to three hours until the water reduces to only one third of the original amount. Then, you use a filter to remove the herbal residues.

Patient: I see. Should I drink all the herbal juice all at once?

Doctor: No. It lasts for three times.

Patient: Anything else that I should pay attention to?

Doctor: Oh, yes the ginseng in the formula should be sliced and decocted separately.

Patient: I see some medicines are of small bits. Should I put them in a bag or something?

Doctor: Yes, very small substances such as powders, seeds and some flowers should be wrapped in a small bag. Plus, *Bohe*(peppermint) should be placed into concoction just before the cooking process is completed.

Patient: It's so complicated a process, but I have taken it down. Doctor, and thank you for your instruction.

Doctor: You are welcome.

IV Oral Practice

Situational Dialogues

Situation 1

Suppose you are an exporter of Chinese herbs in a trade fair. A foreigner shows great interest in these herbs. To you, it is a wonderful chance to introduce and promote your products. Hence, you are going to introduce some traditional Chinese drugs to your customer. You can introduce these drugs from their names, effects, color, even some legends related to them.

Situation 2

Jack has been suffering from stomachache for a long time and one day he went to a TCM clinic and the doctor prescribed him a Chinese herbal formula. But he has has never decocted any Chinese herbs, so he went to a nurse for help. Try to make up a dialogue between Jack and the nurse.

Situation 3

Lily is recently troubled by her weight. Li Lei suggests using Chinese herbs to lose weight instead of taking chemical medicine. Chinese herbs come from the nature, and this is a healthy way for weight loss. TCM holds that obesity is generally caused by *qi* deficiency and endocrine disorders.

The following is a recommended recipe:

Ingredients:

Sangye (Folium Mori) 10g
Baihe (Bulbus Lilii) 10g
Sangshen (Mulberry Fruit) 10g
Tiandong (Radix Asparagi) 10g
Juemingzi (Cassia Seed) 10g
Fanxieye (Folium Sennae) 10g

How to make it

Put these herbs in boiling water and soak them for 3~5 minutes. Take the brew in the morning and the evening. This recipe can be recycled for 2 days, or else you will use the new herbs. Check the effect one week later.

Principle of weight loss: this recipe can remove excess oil from the body and eliminate toxins. After using it for a while, you will feel relaxed.

Precaution: You needn't to go on diet, but note that you shouldn't eat spicy food. After stopping taking it, avoid overeating, otherwise you will gain weight again. This formula may cause mild diarrhea, which is normal.

Story Retelling

Cue Words

(1) 陈皮   dried orange peel
(2) 药丸   pill
(3) 风寒咳嗽   cough due to wind-cold evil
(4) 瓤   flesh, pulp

华佗发现陈皮

这年，华佗外出行医，一日他乘船去柴桑（今江西九江），船进入赣江时，华佗突遭风寒，身上发热，咳嗽不止，口也很干。他忙打开包袱找起药丸来，但治风寒咳嗽的药丸已没有了。正好此时船过三湖，只见岸上桔树成林，红桔累累。华佗想，药丸没了，就想买点桔子吃，至少也能解渴，便叫船夫靠岸，上去买了一筐桔子，回到船上，他连皮带瓤一连吃了好几个。

到了晚上，华佗忽感咳嗽好多了。他感到奇怪：自己没吃药，咳嗽怎好些了呢？他想起白天吃了不少桔子，难道桔子能治咳嗽？第二天，船上的两个船夫也染上感冒，咳嗽起来，华佗便拿出桔子给他们吃。

谁料，两个船夫吃后，一个咳嗽止了，一个却仍咳个不停，华佗挺纳闷，问了才知道，止住咳的一个也是将桔子连皮带瓤一起吃，而无效的一个是只吃桔瓤没吃桔皮。华佗禁不住道："莫非桔皮可止咳？"

之后一路上，华佗每次吃桔子时，都把桔皮留下。数月后，华佗行医归来，发现那些桔皮都风干了，他不知道风干的桔皮是否还有药用。这天，正好有人患伤风咳嗽前来就诊，华佗便把风干的桔皮煎水让病人服用，没想到效果更佳，华佗这才发觉"陈"皮比"鲜"皮更好。

就这样，华佗发现了陈皮。从此，陈皮成了一种不错的中药材。

Group Task

Task 1

Most of the Chinese medicinal herbs come from plants. The places of origin and acquisition time are important factors in terms of quality and effectiveness. Chinese ancient doctors attached great importance to this crucial aspect and have accumulated rich experience in practice. Modern researchers also point out that places of production and acquisition time for herbal medicine determine the effective component in Chinese herbs. Work in groups to find some examples of genuine regional Chinese medicinal herbs and their properties and functions.

Task 2

The naming of traditional Chinese herbs is interesting. Many herbs are named out of their unique physical appearance. For example, *Niuxi* (Radix cyathulaeseuachyranthis), "cow's knees" which has big joints that might look like cow knees; *Baimuer* (Fructificatio tremellae fuciformis), "white wood ear" which is white and resembles an ear; *Gouji* (Rhizoma cibotii), "dog spine" which resembles the spine of a dog.

Can you illustrate others methods of giving names to Chinese herbs?

Task 3

In people's daily life, there are many kinds of commonly-used herbs. You are asked to introduce a kind of herb with detailed information, including place of origin, possible relative stories, properties and tastes, functions, and administration methods.

Reading and Question Answering

Passage 1

Goji Berry Lovers Around the World Wolf Down China's Superfood

Goji berries are found all over China, from flasks of tea in offices through breakfast gruel to braised meat broths in Chinese kitchens. Chinese people like to eat them raw, in tea or soups. Overseas fans make smoothies, salads and cakes. The berries can also be ingredients for facial masks, vitamin tablets and beer.

Also known as the wolfberry, the goji berry and its products are increasingly sought after overseas. Northwest China's Ningxia Hui Autonomous Region grows vast quantities of *Goji* berries, over 60,000 hectares of them. And annual production tops 180,000 tons. Last year, exports reached 7,300 tons, according to data from the regional forestry administration.

"Exports of *Goji* berries and products are growing by about 20 percent each year," said Chen Jianhua, deputy head of the administration.

"A kilogram of *Goji* berries sells for only 100 yuan ($16). The berries themselves do not bring much profit, but downstream products can be very profitable," explained Qiao Changsheng, executive chairman of the Ningxia Qiyuantang Goji Industrial Innovation Institute.

China's *Goji* berry history dates back thousands of years. In ancient traditional Chinese medicine, its functions included protecting the liver, improving eyesight and conserving strength.

China has 133,000 hectares of *Goji* berries, mainly in the northwestern provinces. Ningxia has established standard farming techniques to control the use of pesticides, improve the qualities of the berries and develop new products, said Chen. *Goji* products from Ningxia are exported to 30 countries and regions including US, European Union, Japan and Australia.

Passage 2

TCM Take on Swine Flu-It's Pathogenic Heat, Cold and Damp

Swine flu, or more accurately A(H1N1) flu, has alerted people around the world and in China where many people take anti-viral medication to prevent catching flu.

TCM practitioners urge people to take the standard precautions-primarily frequent hand washing, airing of rooms. If you feel sick, see a doctor.

TCM regards and treats ailments as energy imbalances. It does not have a "germ theory of disease" but perceives pathogens as environmental factors such as pathogenic heat, cold, wind and damp.

Improving one's healthy energy (*qi*) and boosting immunity can help defending against the flu, according Dr Wu Yingen, a member of the Shanghai Expert Panel on Preventing and Controlling A(H1N1) flu. He is the chief physician of Longhua Hospital attached to Shanghai University of TCM.

"The flu is likely caused by invasion of pathogenic heat, pathogenic cold and pathogenic dampness, according to its different symptoms," says Dr Wu.

Sore throat and fever suggest pathogenic heat, aches and pains suggest pathogenic cold, while diarrhea and stomachache indicate pathogenic damp, he says.

To treat patients with respiratory symptoms, herbs like *Zhimahuang* (Chinese ephedra) and *Chaihu* (Chinese thorowax) are recommended. There are also effective Chinese patent drugs including *Banlangen Chongji* (radix isatidis medicinal granules), *Shuanghuanglian* (oral liquid composed of honeysuckle, baikal skullcap root and forsythia), and *Zheng chaihu yin keli* (Chinese thorowax granules).

To relieve digestive system symptoms, TCM recommends herbs like *Gegen* (radix puerariae) and ageratum. People can take patent drugs such as *Huoxiang zhengqi zhiji* (ageratum oral liquid) and *Gegenqinlian* (pills composed of radix puerariae, baikal skullcap root, coptis root and liquorice).

For those with high fever, chest congestion, irritability and breathing problems, TCM recommends patent drugs like *Qingkailing* pills and *Angong niuhuangwan*, mainly composed of herbs like cow-bezoar, cornu bubali, musk and baikal skullcap root.

These medicines are effective in treating other kinds of flu, according to Dr Wu. They only treat symptoms, however, and do not prevent people from catching flu.

To prevent A(H1N1) flu, some people turn to medicines like anti-viral oral liquid, even though they are completely healthy. But this is unnecessary and unhelpful because it doesn't work and extensive self-dosing can cause drug-resistance and make future treatment difficult.

TCM drugs like radix isatidis medicinal granules can help relieve symptoms, but don't prevent this new flu or other flus, says Dr Wu.

"You cannot prevent catching flu by taking anti-viral medication as the flu virus mutates so quickly," says Dr Wu. Medication must be specific to the virus. "Strengthening your healthy energy, in other words, improving your immunity can help fight the invasion of pathogenic energies that cause flu."

Questions

(1) What are the medicinal functions of *Goji* berry?

(2) What are the various ways that people eat *Goji* berry ?

(3) Do you know any effective herbal medicine for treating pandemic flu?

(4) Share your personal experience of using medicinal herbs.

V Creative Oral Activity

Activity 1

You are a student majoring in Chinese medicine in Jiangxi University of Chinese Medicine. One day, a class of elementary students came to *Shennong* Garden for a field trip. You were asked to be the guide of those students and required to introduce the Chinese herbs in *Shennong* Garden in a simple and clear way. Please make up a dialogue based on the given situation.

Activity 2

Chinese people are very good at making herbal tea in order to maintain health, as they know clearly the properties of different medicinal herbs and make different combinations of herbs in various seasons.

In summer, people make tea that is cooling and refreshing with healing properties such as detoxing and calming. A typical example is *Suan Mei Tang* (syrup of plum), consisting of ingredients like black plum, hawthorn, tangerine peel, osmanthus fragrans, licorice, rock sugar, etc. It is regarded as a traditional summer drink to relieve summer-heat in China and once served as a royal drink, because it has the function of dispelling heat and producing coolness, relieving cough and removing phlegm, producing saliva and quench thirst.

Can you give more examples of herbal tea in different seasons and different parts of China, including the ingredients, brewing process and functions of the tea?

References

［1］曹丽娅，李远方.中医英语视听说［M］.青岛：中国海洋大学出版社，2014.

［2］刘明，（美）郝吉顺.中医英语基础教程［M］.上海：复旦大学出版社，2013.

［3］孙文钟.实用中医汉语：口语基础篇［M］.北京：外语教学与研究出版社，2009.

［4］梁琦慧，邹德芳.医学英语口语教程［M］.上海：复旦大学出版社，2011.

［5］李照国，张庆荣.中医英语［M］.上海：上海科学技术出版社，2013.

［6］王文秀，贾轶群，王颖.英汉对照中医英语会话［M］.北京：人民卫生出版社，2014.